Praise for *The Empty Medicine Cabinet*

"This wonderful book shows you that the most powerful medicines are on your plate. The foods you eat every day have the power to prevent illness and to even reverse it. This book will be your guide to unlocking this power. And all the "side effects" are good ones: Easy weight loss, lower cholesterol, and a longer life."

—Neal Barnard, MD
President of Physicians Committee for Responsible Medicine
Author of *Power Foods for the Brain*

"This book is unique in that Dustin Rudolph offers a pharmacist's perspective and experience—working with doctors, many of whom over-prescribe medicines that provide little benefit to most patients. His story, experiences, and the stories of others he includes in his book are great examples of how a plant-based diet can turn even an extremely ill person's life around. The book proves that almost everyone benefits from adopting a plant-based diet, and health improvement is faster and better than with drug treatment."

—Pamela A. Popper, PhD, ND
Executive Director of The Wellness Forum
Author of *Food Over Medicine*

"Do you want to take charge of your health? Read this outstanding book and learn how to take advantage of the enormous healing powers of excellent nutrition. Your body will thank you for the rest of your life."

—John Robbins
President of The Food Revolution Network
Author of *Diet for a New America* and *The Food Revolution*

"Dustin Rudolph is a renegade pharmacist who knows from experience that health can't be ordered from a prescription pad. Instead, he's given us an engaging and accessible guide to a scientifically proven way of eating and living that hedges our bets against disease—and does it deliciously."

—Victoria Moran
  Author of *Main Street Vegan*

"Instead of being a pharmacist pushing pills, Dustin is a "farm assist" pushing plants. Most people are illiterate when it comes to the power of a whole foods, plant-based diet to prevent, halt, and even reverse the majority of chronic Western disease. Read this compellingly clear and concise book from a perspective we've never seen before and become literate and take back your health!"

—Rip Esselstyn
  Author of *The Engine 2 Diet* and *My Beef with Meat*

"Learn how to take charge of your own health—from an industry insider who has learned that our outrageously ineffective healthcare system is really a 'disease management' system. A man of great integrity, this enlightened Doctor of Pharmacy teaches his patients how to eliminate their pills."

—J. Morris Hicks
  Speaker, Consultant, Author of *Healthy Eating, Healthy World*
  International Blogger at hpjmh.com

"Just imagine, a book by a pharmacist who dares to tell the truth about prescription drugs! A major highlight among many was an explanation of the mismanagement of type 2 diabetes. It's not just the wrong diet, it's not just insulin resistance, it's another factor that no one else will tell you about—because they don't know! But, bottom line, a complete reversal! With each chapter and each case history, I'm cheering as I read along. This guy's got it right! My biggest fear is that it won't be read by those so closed-minded that they won't even entertain the possibility of 'an empty medicine cabinet.' Don't you dare be one of those!"

—Ruth Heidrich, PhD
  Ironman Triathlete
  Author of *A Race for Life*, *Senior Fitness*, and *Lifelong Running*

"Who better than a pharmacist, deeply schooled in the complexities of the human body, to let you know the real story about treating illness symptoms with drugs vs. curing disease with diet? *The Empty Medicine Cabinet* is an easy-to-read yet in-depth review of what science has discovered about food and disease. You will discover dangers of medications that big drug companies don't want you to know. Once you learn how to prevent and often reverse disease with simple lifestyle changes, you can boost your health and keep your dollars in your own wallet, not the health care industry's bank account. This book goes on to give you many practical tips on starting and maintaining a plant-based diet, including delicious recipes for meals and snacks. Dustin Rudolph gives you all the facts you need with no sugar-coating, so you can regain the health that you deserve to enjoy."

—Janice Stanger, PhD
Author of *The Perfect Formula Diet*

"After an "undercover" decade and a half in the world of prescription drugs, renegade plant-based pharmacist Dustin Rudolph reveals the truth about the pills we pop every day: they're expensive, often ineffective, and largely unnecessary. In a friendly and conversational style, Rudolph shares the science that Big Pharma spends millions trying to discredit. That simple everyday foods can heal more quickly, profoundly, and broadly than any pill. Read *The Empty Medicine Cabinet* immediately, and buy a copy for your doctor and pharmacist while you're at it. This revolutionary, common-sense information can save thousands of lives a year."

—Howard Jacobson, PhD
Contributing author to *WHOLE: Rethinking the Science of Nutrition*

"Dustin Rudolph has compiled a deeply informed, definitive guide detailing the multiple health problems presented by our modern Western diet – and underscoring the simple solution: a whole foods, plant-based food plan. Reader-friendly and exhaustive, *The Empty Medicine Cabinet* has become a trusted resource on my reference bookshelf. Finally, a pharmacist you can trust."

—Lani Muelrath, MA
Author of *The Plant-Based Journey* and *Fit Quickies*

"Dustin Rudolph provides an empowering exploration of pharm versus food from the unique perspective of a Doctor of Pharmacy, and an expert in nutrition and lifestyle medicine. Informative, inspiring, and insightful, *The Empty Medicine Cabinet* is a must-read."

—Brenda Davis, RD
Author of *Becoming Vegan, Express Addition: The Everyday Guide to Plant-Based Nutrition*

THE **EMPTY** **MEDICINE** **C**A**BINET**

The Pharmacist's Guide

to the Hidden Danger of Drugs

and the Healing Powers of Food

Dustin Rudolph, PharmD

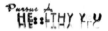

Copyright © 2014 by Dustin L. Rudolph, PharmD

First trade paperback edition 2014

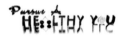

Pursue A Healthy You, LLC
39650 U.S. Highway 19 N. Ste. 736
Tarpon Springs, FL 34689

ISBN 978-0-9915490-1-6

Library of Congress Control Number: 2014906776

Cover design by Wandita Cindyani

This book is dedicated to all individuals suffering from a chronic disease, who've been told that medications and modern medicine are your only hope to regaining optimal health. It is my sincere intention for this message of healing through the application of simple lifestyle changes to truly resonate with you, allowing you to understand that you are not an unfortunate victim of inherited genetic factors or other uncontrollable circumstances.

Contents

Part III – Delicious Eats and Cool Treats

Introduction

Your decision to pick up this book is the first and greatest step toward improving your overall health and well-being. You are about to enter a world where you take back control of your own destiny. Instead of relying on the status quo of our current medical system to get you back on your feet and feeling great, I will show you how to prevent or reverse some of the most common medical problems we all encounter.

Too often, people in our society feel completely dependent on their doctors and other healthcare practitioners to provide them with the answers and treatments they're looking for. They desperately seek to reclaim the active lives they once led before succumbing to their illness. More often than not, they are left feeling discouraged, frustrated, and hopeless as yet another pill, fancy procedure, or expensive device has left them in the same old predicament—sick and worn out. I'm here to tell you that it doesn't have to be this way and that you deserve better.

I've been a practicing pharmacist in our current healthcare system for well over a decade now. I've worked in both the retail pharmacy and inpatient hospital settings. My eyes have been opened to a great deal of pain and suffering during this time. I've seen patients burdened with an array of chronic illnesses that include cardiovascular disease, obesity, diabetes, cancer, arthritis, osteoporosis, and autoimmune disorders such as lupus, migraine headaches, dementia, asthma, allergies, and many more.

Even though many of the patients I've seen have suffered from various diseases, they've all shared one thing in common—they keep coming back for more treatment. If they keep coming back for more treatment, then that means one thing—they're still sick and worn out.

It's not uncommon for me to see patients like the following in my everyday duties as a hospital pharmacist:

Case #1: A fifty-three-year-old woman is admitted directly from her doctor's office complaining of severe abdominal pain. Betty is extremely weak, confused, and hasn't had much of an appetite lately even though she's been drinking water like it's going out of style. Her doctor checked her blood sugar at the office and found it was five times the normal level. Up to this point Betty has no history of diabetes but is currently taking four other medications for various reasons—Synthroid for thyroid disease, Prilosec for acid reflux, Prozac for depression, and a diuretic for high blood pressure. Betty was also complaining of not being able to sleep well since starting on Prozac.

After spending one day in the intensive care unit and four days total in the hospital, Betty is finally well enough to go home. Her blood sugar is back to normal but not without the help of more medication. She's now leaving with five additional medications—metformin, glyburide, and insulin shots for her new diagnosis of diabetes, lisinopril to help protect her kidneys since she's now diabetic, and Ambien to help counteract the insomnia caused by Prozac. Betty will have to check her blood sugars a minimum of four times a day at home and will sadly become a "regular" around the hospital due to continued complications of her diabetes.

Case #2: Jim, age fifty-nine, is rushed to the emergency room with crushing chest pain. He has never had a heart attack before this but has been flirting with disaster over the past decade because he's developed some bad habits in his later years, such as not exercising and eating out a lot. His doctor put him on Lipitor for his cholesterol seven years ago, and since then he's had three additional drugs added to the list—Norvasc and Lasix for high blood pressure and Viagra for erectile dysfunction.

After a crazy initial ten minutes in the ER, Jim is stabilized and then whisked to the cath lab to have a stent placed in one of his coronary arteries. Three days go by before Jim is finally well enough to go home but not before having four more medications added to his daily regimen. This makes eight now with the new drugs being Coreg and Vasotec for blood pressure along with Plavix and aspirin to thin his blood.

Although Jim's life was saved this time, he leaves the hospital with a false sense of security that his new stent and medication regimen will protect him from any future heart attacks. The worst is not over, however. Little does he know that in fourteen months he'll be readmitted to the hospital with the very same problem. This time two more stents are required to open up completely clogged arteries surrounding his heart.

In an age where technology and all that it has to offer has become so readily available in the modern medical system, why are we seeing cases like these over and over again? Never before have we had more medications, state-of-the-art equipment, or cutting-edge procedures available to us than we do today.

The statistics can be mind-boggling when you look at them. Over four billion prescriptions were filled in the United States in 2011, and approximately three-fourths of all visits to the doctor involved drug therapy.[1,2] Over 850,000 coronary angioplasties and more than 250,000 open heart surgeries were performed in 2008 in the United States.[3] We spent over $2.7 trillion on healthcare in the U.S. in 2011 alone, which is nearly double per person what other developed nations spend on their citizens.[4]

Yet, despite these numbers Americans are growing fatter and getting sicker by the day. Everyone seems to be looking for that one simple fix that will make their problems vanish overnight. In spite of all the well-meaning intentions of both doctors and patients, none of these modern remedies seems to work. Something has definitely gone wrong.

All of this seems to raise more questions than answers for both patients and doctors. It's easy to give up hope and just accept the fact that you're destined to spend the last two to four decades of your life taking a handful of pills and going from one doctor to the next in search of answers. However, the answers to these tough questions are better served by less medical care, not more, as you will soon find out. This was best put into words by one of our country's most famous founding fathers when Benjamin Franklin said, "Nothing is more fatal to health than an over care of it."

It's as if Benjamin Franklin had a crystal ball and was looking into the twenty-first century. After reading this book you'll have a clear understanding of exactly why "over care" may be so fatal.

In my daily duties as a pharmacist it's not uncommon for me to see a patient be put on one drug to counteract the adverse effects of another. Before you know it, this patient has a list of medications that reaches into the double digits and monthly co-pays that force them to re-evaluate their family budget. Instead of

> **Your key to success comes in the form of a grocery list and not a prescription.**

feeling better, patients typically feel worse or, at best, the same as before they started. So how do we go from feeling broke, sick, and helpless to feeling robust, healthy, and empowered?

We will explore this solution together as this book reveals the power of plant-based nutrition. Your key to success comes in the form of a grocery list and not a prescription. This program is not the latest fad or just another one of those diets failing to live up to infomercial hype but rather a lifestyle program that has been proven to be the most effective way to achieve optimal health while permanently reaching your ideal weight at the same time.

If you've tried every diet known to man and none of them has worked, don't despair. This program has worked for thousands of patients and will work for you too. The information I will give you is backed by an array of scientific evidence that has been published over the last several decades in many highly respected scientific and medical journals. I will teach you the same strategies used, with unrivaled success, by leading experts and clinicians in the field of medicine. The results you will see, and the transformation you experience, will make you wonder why our current medical system hasn't given these strategies the emphasis they deserve.

As the saying goes—the proof is in the pudding—but it's a different kind of pudding both figuratively and literally, and it's starting to grab the attention of the mainstream media. Talk shows, news broadcasts, print media, and even documentaries are now starting to share this life-saving message as our nation tries to find a way to tackle the growing healthcare crisis.

Significant hurdles remain, though, and you'll learn how vested corporate and political interests are attempting to keep this information from reaching the masses. As you are aware, the public's best interests are not always well served by those in a position of power. There is no doubt that our most pressing issues today rarely find a satisfactory outcome because of the sheer magnitude of special interest money floating around within the circles of the privileged few at the top. Prime examples of this type of malfeasance are our healthcare and food industries.

You will soon come to understand the critical need for a grassroots movement to carry a different message forward for the betterment of all—a message that inspires hope and produces results in the form of increased health and happiness for individuals throughout our nation, whether it is in the small communities of the Midwest or the sprawling urban suburbs of the Northeast. We all deserve a life where we're not just living longer but living better with a higher quality of life well into our eighties and nineties.

I invite you to join me as I unveil the secrets to health, longevity, and ultimately greater happiness as you find yourself living a lifestyle devoid of chronic illness, free of prescription medications, and full of energy. This program can change your life as it has changed mine. I live by these same principles and have helped many others get the most out of their lives because these methods work.

Through my experience as a pharmacist, I have witnessed all that conventional medicine has to offer. There are many things physicians, surgeons, and medicine can do that have no substitute. Healthy lifestyles cannot fix a broken leg or put an end to a terrifying grand mal seizure. Nor can eating healthy foods and exercising cure a life-threatening case of pneumonia. This is not a book of holistic medicine full of "natural" powders, potions, and pills.

Instead, what you will learn is that by following the steps I set out for you, you and your family will enjoy a longer and healthier life. A life less likely to be encumbered by the many preventable diseases that plague humanity. I know of no better way to achieve these goals and end the current healthcare crisis in America than by following these principles. Come now and give yourself a brand new start at life as you embark on a promising future of health and prosperity laid out here in *The Empty Medicine Cabinet*.

Part I

Paving the Way to Better Overall Health

Avoid the Pill Trap

*"The marvelous pharmacy that was designed by
nature and placed into our being by the universal
architect produces most of the medicines we need."*
—NORMAN COUSINS

It was one of those picture-perfect summer mornings as my family made our way up the narrow dirt road leading to my grandfather's small farm in southeast, rural Montana. My grandpa's farm was every young boy's dream. It was a place where little boys could do grown-up things without getting into trouble from nosy neighbors or the local sheriff's deputy patrolling the quiet residential streets of the city.

We'd start the day with a trip to the chicken coop to gather eggs from my grandfather's prize brood of hens. He'd always boast about how his chickens were the only chickens around that would naturally lay colored eggs. He called these birds his "Easter chickens," and the bottom of their nests would greet him every morning lined with light shades of brown, green, and golden yellow eggs.

Next, we were off to my favorite part of visiting grandpa on his farm— driving the tractor! Grandpa would hoist me up onto his big, blue antiquated

Ford. With him seated behind me, I would grab hold of the mammoth steering wheel as we set out to plow his boundless fields of potatoes and corn. Grandpa had four acres of potato fields, another acre of corn, and two large vegetable gardens. We'd work all day in these fields and then gather back at his house to have a huge cookout filled with steaks, hamburgers, fried potato cuts, and corn on the cob dripping with melted butter. We'd top it all off with a big bowl of hand-cranked vanilla ice cream. A perfect ending for a hot summer day! Those were the times, but little did I know how precious these memories would be as the years passed by.

It was New Year's Eve 1993 when we got the call. My Grandpa Rudy had finally lost his battle with heart disease and diabetes. He had passed away at the age of seventy-six. He had spent the previous three to four years in and out of the VA hospital trying to overcome the debilitating effects of these two chronic medical conditions. My grandpa had followed in the footsteps of his father who had died of a massive heart attack at fifty-nine.

My grandfather never smoked cigarettes, rarely consumed alcohol, and had been extremely active throughout his life. He spent much of his career doing hard manual labor in the oil fields. He was also involved with the Boy Scouts in his spare time. His vigorous lifestyle was certainly a big part of why he had remained so strong and healthy into his late sixties.

Another striking feature about my grandfather's life was that he ate what many would consider a well-balanced diet. Processed food—such as frozen dinners, packaged goods, or fast food—weren't widely available for most of his life, and even when they did arrive in the latter part of the twentieth century, he never took a liking to them. Instead, he stuck to his daily meat and potatoes diet, along with a good helping of fresh vegetables. His normal meal is what most people would consider the classic All-American diet—high-quality protein, real potatoes, and a healthy serving of colorful vegetables. Despite eating a "normal" diet, or perhaps because of it, he couldn't escape the consequences of two of the top ten killer diseases in America.

The last eight years of my grandfather's life were spent in a gradual state of declining health. He was diagnosed with type 2 diabetes and became dependent on numerous shots of insulin throughout the day. He also took a handful of medications, both morning and night, to combat his heart condition. He gradually became physically unable to do what he had always loved—working on his farm—and would eventually have to move into town in order to be cared for.

When he finally passed, his frail body, diminished frame, and sunken eyes were a far cry from the confident, strong, pot-bellied man I had visited in my childhood days. I was a sophomore in high school at the time of my

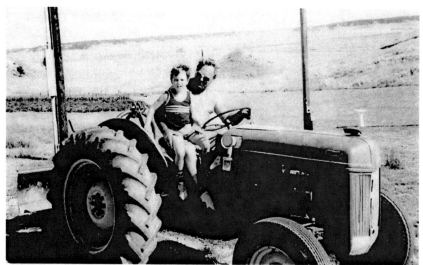
My grandfather and me on his farm in Montana.

grandfather's death and had dreams of becoming a pharmacist. I wanted to help people just like him, so they could live longer and healthier lives. My grandfather never got the opportunity to see me accomplish my dream, nor did he get the chance to know my two younger brothers as they grew up and pursued dreams of their own. Preventable medical conditions had prematurely taken his life.

This story is not unique today. I'm sure you can relate through your own experience or through happenings with your family. All too often, we become complacent and develop habits that don't fit well with our long-term interests. We sleep too little, drink too much, and eat the wrong types of foods. Eventually, weight gain and fatigue set in while the initial signs of serious medical conditions pop up—high blood pressure, high cholesterol, elevated blood sugar levels, and more. Because we can't see or feel these silent "red flags," we continue unhealthy behaviors without ever giving much thought to the trap we're setting for ourselves.

A routine trip to the doctor for an annual checkup reveals the truth—a less than clean bill of health. This leads to the familiar talk with the doctor about diet and exercise. While many physicians have good intentions, they've been shuffled through an educational system that puts little or no emphasis on lifestyle medicine (that is, the practice of using nutrition, exercise, and other healthy habits to prevent and reverse chronic diseases).

That's why our healthcare practitioners work with what they've learned, dispensing advice outlined by prominent organizations such as the American Diabetes Association, American Cancer Society, and American Heart

Association. These recommendations include staying away from processed foods, eating leaner meats, switching to low-fat dairy products, and including plenty of fruits and vegetables in our diet. Sound advice to many.

Follow-up visits to the doctor almost always bring feelings of frustration and disappointment. Your numbers aren't hitting the mark, and the aches and pains aren't going away. You're concerned and so is your physician because ignoring these problems is only going to make matters worse. You've already tried diet and exercise and that didn't work. So both you and your doctor resort to the fact that your medical condition is probably just due to family history or bad "genes." Next, the prescription pad comes out and the process repeats itself year after year after year.

This is the status quo for how we conduct business in our current healthcare system. However, it doesn't have to be this way. There is a better way! It involves approaching disease and sickness at its foundation instead of covering up the symptoms with medications and risky procedures. By using lifestyle medicine we address the root causes of disease instead of tackling the symptoms. This approach is far more effective, safer, and less costly than conventional medicine, and, most importantly—it works!

Lifestyle medicine doesn't get all the media attention and hype that modern medicine gets because, quite frankly, it's not a good business model for generating profits. As a patient, you're only an asset to Big Healthcare if you linger between perfectly healthy and dead. Having a chronic disease requires continuous medical care involving costly follow-up visits, medications, and many different surgeries and procedures over time. This is great news for the pharmaceutical industry, medical supply companies, and healthcare organizations because you're now a customer for life. Lifestyle medicine prevents you from being in this position, putting you back in control of your own destiny.

> As a patient, you're only an asset to Big Healthcare if you linger between perfectly healthy and dead.

Before I researched lifestyle medicine, I was of the belief that conventional medicine, with its state-of-the-art treatments, was the only responsible and effective way to treat the assortment of chronic diseases we see today. Having been instructed in the same educational system as your doctor, I came to understand that the power of the prescription pad was ingrained into my head. There was a pill for everything, and as a pharmacist I had embraced the pill-popping nation that we'd become. The numbers tell a scary story:

- In 2010, we spent $307 billion on prescription medications in the U.S. with an average of nearly thirteen prescriptions being dispensed for every man, woman, and child.[1]
- Cardiovascular disease remains the number one killer worldwide and has been the leading cause of death in the United States since 1921.[2,3]
- Type 2 diabetes now affects over 25 million people in America with projections estimated to rise above 86 million by 2050.[4,5]
- Cancer, the second leading cause of death in the U.S., is still running rampant in our country, even after spending billions of dollars attempting to "find a cure." The four most common types of cancer—prostate, breast, lung, and colorectal—can often be prevented simply by making smarter choices in how we eat and by avoiding the use of tobacco.[6]

These are not promising figures and we need to embrace a different approach if we wish to live a longer, healthier, and higher quality of life. To do this, our most powerful tool comes in the form of adopting a whole foods, plant-based lifestyle. This approach has been used by several physicians, whom you will come to know in the following chapters, as a foundation for their medical practices. They have seen overwhelming success rates, with their patients often achieving a disease-free life without the need for prescription medications. Had I known this information before my grandfather's death, there is no doubt I could've helped him live longer. He might have even been able to see his grandchildren fulfill their dreams.

This is the kind of life I want for you—to see your grandchildren and great grandchildren fulfill their dreams. My hope is that by embracing the guidelines in the upcoming chapters, you will escape the pill trap so many fail to escape as they pass through their middle years. I know of no better way to do this than to share the benefits a plant-based lifestyle has to offer. This lifestyle change is so effective that I must warn you now, if you are currently taking medications, you will need to consult your doctor, as in all likelihood, some or all of your medications may need to be adjusted or eventually eliminated altogether. If you are not currently taking medications, I'm confident the chance of your needing them after adopting this program is remarkably small. Brace yourself, for you are about to learn how to avoid *the pill trap*!

Lose Weight, Gain Health, Eat as Much as You Want

"The best diet is the one you don't know you're on."
—BRIAN WANSINK

I t's everywhere you look these days—extra body fat packed onto our waistlines, butts, thighs, hips, arms, and even our chins. Nobody wants the extra baggage that is inevitably added over the years, but both short- and long-term weight loss can seem like trying to win the $500-million Powerball. No matter what combination of diets, exercise regimens, or supplements you try, it's just not enough to beat the odds and cash in on the winning ticket.

The total amount of weight that America has been packing on in recent years is almost unimaginable. David Satcher, the U.S. Surgeon General in 2001, stated in the *F as in Fat* report that over the past decade America has gained over 4.5 billion extra pounds![1] This works out to be approximately the same amount of weight that a fleet of over 11,250 Boeing 747's would weigh before being loaded down with passengers and their luggage. It's no wonder the airlines are charging extra fees for those of us taking up more than our fair share of an assigned seat.

With more than two-thirds of adults and one of every three children considered overweight or obese in America, we have a major healthcare crisis taking place, and it isn't showing any signs of slowing down. The Surgeon General's *F as in Fat* report is aimed at raising awareness and bringing action to combat the obesity epidemic in America.

The classification of being obese is defined as having a body mass index (BMI) of greater than 30, while a classification of being overweight is defined as having a BMI of greater than 25. In the 2011 report, only one state in the U.S. had an obesity rate of less than 20 percent and that state was Colorado. Twelve states actually had an obesity rate of greater than 30 percent. Compare that to twenty years ago when not a single state had an obesity rate of more than 15 percent. We've come a long way in those two decades, but it certainly isn't in the right direction. Our waistlines are literally killing us.

The good news is this weight gain doesn't have to happen to you. Whether you're looking to lose weight now or just want to avoid putting on any extra pounds, you'll have no problem accomplishing this by adopting the same approach that has worked for thousands of others in the past. This approach is a whole foods, plant-based lifestyle, described in detail in chapter 9. The best part about this approach is that you won't have to sacrifice taste, and, better yet, you'll *never, ever* have to count calories again.

You're probably thinking to yourself right about now that this sounds too good to be true. Well, it's not. Research performed by Joel Fuhrman, MD, provides evidence showing how much more enjoyable eating this way really can be. While following his high-nutrient, plant-based diet, individuals actually had less hunger discomfort and enjoyed the act of eating more than they had previously on their normal diets.[2] This new way of eating is also more beneficial for your overall health and it's exactly what our country needs as the obesity epidemic is literally transforming us into one of the sickest nations on the face of the planet.

Health Risks of Excess Weight

All this extra weight comes at a major price to those who are lugging it around. Being overweight or obese increases your risk for over twenty different chronic diseases. These conditions include many of the common diseases listed in the top ten leading causes of death, such as heart disease and stroke. It also consists of some less common disorders such as osteoarthritis and sleep apnea that still cause a lot of unnecessary pain and suffering for those affected by them.[3] A quick glance at the following shows just how serious a problem being overweight or obese can be:[4-7]

- Of patients with type 2 diabetes, 85 percent are overweight.
- Kidney disease is increased by 83 percent if you're obese and 40 percent if you're overweight.
- Obesity directly causes 75 percent or more of all high blood pressure cases.
- The following health conditions are linked to being overweight or obese:
  - High cholesterol
  - Hypertriglyceridemia
  - Coronary heart disease
  - Strokes
  - Metabolic syndrome
  - Cancer
  - Osteoarthritis
  - Gallstones
  - Infertility
  - Sleep apnea

Being overweight is clearly a detriment to your health and losing excess weight is beneficial for anyone who does so. What's interesting, though, is it's not only the amount of extra weight that poses a health risk to an individual but also where this weight is located on the body that determines a person's increased risk of certain diseases.

Experts at the World Health Organization found that people with higher amounts of fat located around their waistlines—commonly known as belly fat—had a much higher risk of developing cardiovascular disease (including heart disease and stroke) and type 2 diabetes.[8] These individuals also had a higher rate of overall mortality than did overweight individuals without an excess of belly fat. When the panel of experts looked at cancer, they found two of the most common types of cancer, breast and colorectal, were increased in overweight or obese individuals regardless of whether or not the extra weight was stored in the form of abdominal fat or elsewhere in the body.

You can see how important it is to your overall health to maintain a healthy weight. Losing weight can benefit you no matter how it comes off, but if you want to reduce your risk for even more diseases, then losing belly fat should be of high priority to help you steer clear of heart disease, diabetes, and a higher rate of overall death.

You can skip the diet pills though. As a pharmacist who's worked in the retail setting, I've seen numerous overweight patients head straight for the top shelf of the supplement aisle hoping their favorite concoction of weight loss pills will solve all their problems. They don't. These supplements were not designed with your long-term health or weight loss goals in mind. They are short-term gimmicks aimed at draining your wallet. Many of them speed up your metabolism or reduce your appetite, but they do nothing to address the poor nutritional qualities of the Standard American Diet, which causes obesity in the first place.

[The Standard American Diet, fittingly shortened to the acronym SAD, is a nutrient-poor, calorie-rich Western diet consisting of 51 percent carbohydrates, 16 percent protein, and a whopping 33 percent fat.[9]]

Weight loss supplements also have the potential to be highly dangerous. Ephedra-containing products such as Metabolife 356 have reportedly caused serious heart problems including heart attacks, strokes, and even death.[10] Other weight loss formulations such as Hydroxycut have been known to cause liver toxicity in some people. My advice is simple. Steer clear of all diet pills. They'll rob you of your hard-earned money and possibly even your life.

Broken Promises of Conventional Diets

You've most likely heard the phrase "calories in, calories out" when the diet word pops up in conversation with others. This is referring to the simple equation that burning more calories than you consume will inevitably lead to the desired weight loss you're looking for.

Many typical diets abide by this philosophy, and it's how they get a large number of their participants to reach their weight loss goals, at least in the short term. You may have even tried a number of these diets over the years only to find yourself regaining some or all of your original weight back. That's because living this kind of lifestyle is difficult. Most people can't maintain it for any length of time.

As a human being you were not designed to eat a diet that fails to meet your daily energy needs. That's exactly what many of these diets do. They help you calorie count your way into a deficit. They put your body through the unpleasant experience of not getting the calories (and nutrients) it needs in order to function properly on a daily basis. This is the equivalent to filling up your vehicle with only half a tank of gas when going on a long distance trip. It won't take long before you run out of fuel and fail to reach your destination. Instead, you're stuck in the middle of nowhere irritated and crabby because gassing up halfway didn't work.

The same holds true when your body is experiencing signs of hunger throughout the day. It's asking you to pull over and "gas up." By ignoring these signs or only partially fulfilling your natural desire to feed yourself, you're asking your body to complete its daily journey without the proper amount of nourishment to do so. Eventually, most people just give up because their dieting journey becomes an intolerable experience filled with feelings of frustrations and defeat. Instead, they resort to their old ways and continue a destructive cycle of gaining and losing weight year after year without ever reaching their long-term weight loss goals.

Failing on these types of diets is not your fault. They were never designed for permanent weight loss. They were structured for short-term results to make you feel as if you're winning the battle against unwanted weight gain, even though their long-term track record is pitiful at best. Approximately 80 percent of dieters fail to maintain their initial weight loss after one year on calorie-restriction diets.[11] The five-year data aren't much better.

According to a review of over ten long-term weight loss studies, only 15 percent of people were successful at sustaining their initial weight loss after five years.[12] Not surprising, many individuals actually gained more weight back than they originally started with. This is hardly the definition of success. Counting calories doesn't work. It's simply unsustainable for the vast majority of people.

There *is* a better way however. The new approach addresses what your body is really asking for—adequate nutrition that fulfills both the *macro*nutrient and *micro*nutrient needs of your cells and tissues. This approach addresses your body's short- and long-term nutritional needs, while at the same time advocating healthy weight loss. It satisfies your macronutrient requirements by meeting your body's energy needs through ingesting enough calories. It satisfies your micronutrient requirements by the ample consumption of vitamins, minerals, and antioxidants on a regular basis, all of which are vital to long-term health. You're about to learn how this all fits together and why the nutrient density of your food is so critical in achieving optimal health and in maintaining an ideal body weight for decades to come.

Not All Calories Are Created Equal

Contrary to what you might have learned in the past, not all calories are created equal. It turns out that calories from whole, nutrient-rich, plant-based foods are metabolized much more efficiently than calories from animal-based or processed foods. T. Colin Campbell, PhD, a world-renowned nutritional research scientist, discovered this during his career of fifty-plus years investigating the intricate relationships between health and nutrition.

Dr. Campbell explains in his book, *The China Study*, how the process of thermogenesis allows for your body to burn a portion of the calories consumed from plant foods as body heat rather than storing these calories as body fat.[13] This ultimately leads to less weight gain over time. It's also part of the reason why multiple studies have shown that following a plant-based lifestyle over the long term has resulted in slimmer individuals who experience less weight gain than their meat-eating counterparts.[14,15]

Another fascinating detail from Dr. Campbell's research was the observation he made while comparing the traditional diet of a Chinese adult male to the diet of an American adult male eating the Standard American Diet (SAD). The traditional Chinese diet derives approximately 90 percent of its calories from nutrient-rich, plant-based foods. The SAD diet derives less than 5 to 7 percent of its calories from nutrient-rich, plant-based foods.

The findings? On average, the Chinese male consumed 30 percent more calories each day than his American male counterpart. Yet the Chinese male had a BMI that was 25 percent lower than the average American male's BMI.[16] Again, this signifies how great an impact a diet of plant-based, whole foods has on your ability to successfully lose weight and keep it off, permanently.

You might be thinking to yourself, "Now wait a minute. That's because the Chinese have a more active lifestyle than we Americans, and they have an entirely different genetic makeup than we do too." While this may be a valid notion at first thought, Dr. Campbell made it a point to compare a sample of Chinese men who were the least physically active, working in an office job, instead of choosing men who lived the more traditional Chinese lifestyle of putting in a hard day's work on the family farm.

By controlling his sample, he was comparing apples to apples. Both groups of men were leading a sedentary lifestyle. Therefore, physical activity could not be used to explain the differing BMI results. The Chinese men still ended up weighing a fourth less than the American men while eating 30 percent more calories.

What about the differences between the genetic code of the two cultures? Obviously the DNA of the Asian population is different from that of the American population, right? This would explain why the Asian population is much leaner than Americans, wouldn't it?

One might think so, but once again this is not the case. Studies have shown that as first- and second-generation Asians immigrate to the United States and start to adopt our lifestyle and way of eating, they become much more at risk of becoming overweight and obese.[17,18] Third- and fourth-generation Asian Americans who were born on U.S. soil and live their whole lives in America are at even higher risk of becoming overweight and obese.

If genetic differences were really that powerful in protecting one race of people over another, then it sure isn't panning out that way. When our Asian neighbors adopt our SAD diet, full of highly processed and animal-based foods, they start to balloon up in the same fashion as we Americans do.

The same obesity epidemic that the United States is currently experiencing is now spreading across the globe as our culture of fast food, neighborhood coffee joints, packaged convenience foods, and meat and dairy becomes the everyday reality for our neighbors throughout the world. The world is literally eating itself to death now, albeit slowly, as heart disease, stroke, and diabetes spread like wildfire around the world.

The world is literally eating itself to death now.

Many would agree we're eating far too many unhealthy foods today, seeing for the first time our children having a shorter life expectancy than their parents have. The question is how do we stop this and is it too late? Is simply cutting back and eating in moderation enough or does the answer involve making more profound changes that defy common knowledge?

Eating in Moderation vs. Eating for Nutrient Density

Moderation has been a commonplace philosophy endorsed in many typical diet programs. A number of well-known organizations live by these philosophies to help people lose weight and feel good about themselves. However, they fail to take into account the effects of certain foods on one's long-term health and well-being.

When you cookie cut your diet to fit into lower portion sizes and ignore the nutritional value of the food you're eating, then you're attempting to sidestep the laws of biology. No matter how hard you try, it's impossible to outsmart Mother Nature.

Quite literally, thousands of complex interactions are going on inside your body, which are responsible for maintaining a healthy weight.

It's incredibly difficult to achieve long-term weight loss and get the benefits of excellent health without understanding the concept of nutrient density. Your body knows the difference between fiber and salt, vitamins and sugar, and antioxidants and fat, regardless of which foods these nutrients come from or how they end up getting into your stomach.

In the Western culture we eat a diet containing too many macronutrients and not enough micronutrients leading to nutritional deficiencies. Wait, what does that mean?

It means we need to understand the ABC's of food and its nutritional makeup. Dr. Joel Fuhrman explains this topic in detail in his book *Eat For Health* as he describes two main categories of nutrients—macronutrients and micronutrients. They both have an enormous impact on how well the body functions. Understanding their roles will help you make better food choices going forward. By doing so, you not only give yourself the ability to reach your weight loss goals, but you will improve your overall health at the same time.

Macronutrients are the nutrients everybody obsesses over when they think about the nutritional value of their food. Macronutrients are comprised of three main components—fats, carbohydrates, and proteins. They account for most, if not all, of the calories a person consumes in a day. Part of our weight problem in the U.S. is certainly due to an over consumption of too many macronutrients (aka calories). However, this is *not* the only problem. By focusing only on getting too many calories, most people completely disregard the fact that they're not getting enough of some key additional substances. These key substances happen to be fiber and the other main group of nutrients—micronutrients.

Fiber is an important macronutrient belonging to the carbohydrate family. Although it provides little to no calories to the body—due to its lack of absorption—it does play an extremely beneficial role as part of a healthy diet. It provides extra volume (increasing satiety, that's the sense of feeling full), slows the absorption of glucose aiding in controlling blood sugar levels, lowers cholesterol levels and thus reduces heart disease risk, and helps with the passage of food through the digestive tract by improving defecation and alleviating constipation.[19,20]

Fiber is completely absent in all animal-based foods (meat, dairy, and eggs). Therefore, these foods cannot supply the degree of health-promoting benefits fiber-rich, plant-based foods can. It's important that fiber be obtained directly from plant-based foods too. Benefiber and Metamucil are no substitutes! Studies have shown that fiber supplements produce only minor effects when it comes to weight loss compared to fiber obtained directly from food.[21] Fiber from supplements is also devoid of the other critical class of nutrients—micronutrients.

Micronutrients are a group of nutrients far more important to the quality of one's overall health than macronutrients are. Unfortunately, these nutrients are typically left out of the decision making process as many of us fill our grocery carts with foods lacking any sense of nutritional value at all.

Micronutrients do not contain calories. They are the calorie-free portion of food that consists of the following—vitamins, minerals, antioxidants, and thousands of phytochemicals. Micronutrients are vital for growth and development. These nutrients also play a key role in maintaining an ideal, healthy body weight as well.

Micronutrients are almost exclusively found in plant-based, whole foods such as fruits and vegetables and are largely responsible for the bright colors you see in the plant kingdom. By eating fiber-rich, micronutrient-packed foods, you're naturally consuming foods that have fewer calories and more overall volume, which helps you feel fuller sooner. This in turn leads to less weight gain and more weight loss. Processed and animal-based foods, to the contrary, contain a disproportionately small amount of these vital micronutrients and are unable to provide the same weight loss benefits seen with their colorful plant-based counterparts.[22]

Micronutrients also play a critical role in achieving and maintaining an optimal state of health, free of disease and illness. They help reduce blood pressure and cholesterol levels, lower chronic inflammation, and destroy free radicals before damage to the body's DNA can be done.[23] Free radicals are nothing more than unstable molecules that readily attack healthy cells and tissues in the body leading to ill health.

These important functions of micronutrients all lead to a number of welcomed benefits—lower risk of heart disease, fewer cases of autoimmune disorders, and decreased rates of various cancers. Foods that are higher in micronutrients and lower in macronutrients, such as fruits and vegetables, are far more valuable to your body nutritionally speaking because of these health-promoting benefits. As a result, they have earned the distinction of being labeled nutrient-rich or nutrient-dense foods.

The biggest reason we suffer from so many chronic diseases is because of this deficiency in micronutrient-rich food. We've grown up in a culture where long-held beliefs encourage us to consume whatever foods we want as long as we eat in moderation. This has been ingrained into us since we were children. This line of thinking encourages us to continue eating a diet without giving any thought to the nutritional value of what we're eating. We are only reminded of the fact we should eat less of the bad foods.

Unfortunately, by following this train of thought, we end up eating the same calorie-rich foods, largely devoid of micronutrients, but in smaller quantities only to end up under nourishing our bodies day in and day out. As a result, we have a nation of people becoming increasingly frustrated with the concept of dieting because the end results are the same—lack of long-term sustainable weight loss coupled with an epidemic of chronic diseases.

A Look Around the World

If you look at other cultures throughout the world, you'll find that those that have the lowest rates of chronic diseases are the ones whose citizens consume a whole foods, plant-based diet containing little or no meat, dairy, or processed food. Japan has one of the lowest rates of death due to heart disease in the world, and the typical Japanese diet is based on rice and vegetables with only a small amount of fish included.[24] India has one of the lowest rates of cancer deaths in the world, and they eat a predominantly plant-based diet, also with a large amount of rice and vegetables.[25]

Many of the Central American countries (for example, Mexico, El Salvador, and Guatemala) have some of the lowest rates of death due to both cancer and cardiovascular disease in the world.[26] However, don't let the typical menu from a Mexican-American restaurant lead you astray. Traditional diets of these Central Americans are comprised mostly of corn and beans along with generous amounts of fruits and vegetables. They contain only a small amount of meat and dairy. This is a far cry from the fajitas and burritos jam-packed with beef and chicken rolled up into white flour tortillas, deep fried, and smothered with loads of cheese served in most Mexican restaurants in the United States.

As you can see, cultures with a long history of following a plant-based lifestyle fare well when it comes to avoiding the devastating diseases that plague much of the Western world where processed and animal-based foods overwhelm the average dinner plate. We could learn a lot from our world neighbors by taking notice of these larger portions of nutrient-dense, plant-based foods in their diets. We *must* learn a lot from our friends around the globe if we are to move forward and solve our own obesity epidemic and the resulting healthcare crisis in America.

The Truth of the Matter

The truth is there are good foods and bad foods out there. When you nourish your body with good, wholesome plant-based foods and avoid the bad (animal-based, processed, and refined foods), your body will respond amazingly well. To get exceptional results you need to fill your plate with most, if not all, of these nutrient-dense, plant-based foods.

A number of studies have shown superior weight loss results by doing just that rather than resorting to standard conventional diets preaching moderation:[27-29]

- Individuals following a plant-based diet lost three times more weight after one year and four times more weight after two years than those who followed a conventional diet based on the federal government's National Cholesterol Education Program (NCEP) guidelines.
- A review of multiple studies has shown a continual reduction in body mass index (BMI) as someone goes from being a meat eater to consuming no meat at all to consuming no meat, dairy, or eggs in the diet.
- Observational studies indicate that obesity rates are much lower in those who follow a plant-based diet free of meat (0–6%) compared to those eating a conventional diet that includes meat, dairy, and eggs (5–45%).

Counting calories as part of a conventional diet is a flawed and unreliable means to successful weight loss. Achieving and maintaining an ideal, healthy body weight for years or decades to come rests squarely on gaining an understanding of the nutritional value of the foods you eat. By eating foods that promote long-term health and sustainable weight loss, there is no need to worry about how much you are eating, only that you are eating nutrient-rich foods.

The studies contained in this chapter present a clear picture of how powerful plant-based foods can be. The more you include them in your diet, the better results you'll see. A body powered by plants is a body performing at its finest.

Consuming a diet containing 90 percent or more of your calories from these nutrient-dense, plant-based foods will give you the best chance at long-term success. The guidelines contained in chapter 9 will help you understand how to implement a plant-based lifestyle and send you down a sustainable path of health and newfound freedom.

Healthy Hearts

"Open heart surgery is radical. Eating oatmeal
and potatoes is not radical."

—JOHN MCDOUGALL, MD

The most notorious serial killer of the modern day era is not one of infamy like those of the past—Charles Manson, Ted Bundy, or John Wayne Gacy—but rather one that has no voice, no body, and no mind to calculate its own gruesome deed. It's a killer that revels in the spotlight of social acceptance while delivering death to its next victim once every thirty-nine seconds in the United States.

This dreadful monster is better known as cardiovascular disease, and it's the leading cause of death in both the United States and the rest of the world.[1,2] For well over a century, dating back to 1900, heart disease and stroke have combined to kill more Americans every single year than any other cause.[3] The only exception was in 1918 when a worldwide flu pandemic spread across the globe taking an estimated 30 to 50 million lives with it, including well over half a million Americans.[4]

Chances are you either know someone suffering from cardiovascular disease or are battling it yourself. It's a grueling disease that often involves years or even decades of declining health. My paternal grandfather, whom I spoke of earlier, along with my paternal grandmother, have both fallen victim to this disease. I know how it feels to see a loved one suffer from it. Sometimes the feeling of helplessness is more than one can bear. There always seems to be a never-ending series of medical bills, doctor visits, and prescriptions piling up, and for what? Is any of it doing any good? Heart disease never seems to go away—at least that's the general thinking.

Cardiovascular disease is not only preventable but also reversible in the majority of people. With an open mind and a willingness to adopt a whole foods, plant-based lifestyle nearly everyone can overcome this devastating illness. It's happening every day as people take back control of their own health and seek information available in books like this.

How Cardiovascular Disease Develops

The heart serves as the epicenter of the cardiovascular system. It's the main engine that keeps things running and is accompanied by an endless string of arteries, veins, and capillaries all working in unison with one another to deliver the oxygen and nutrients our tissues and cells need in order to function properly.

The enormity of this system is almost unimaginable. It's so large that if all of the blood vessels were laid out end-to-end they would extend for over 60,000 miles.[5] On top of this, the heart beats an average 100,000 times per day delivering roughly 2,000 gallons of blood throughout this network of arteries, veins, and capillaries.

The Anatomy of an Artery

Arteries are the primary blood vessels affected by diseases of the cardiovascular system. They're made up of three main layers. The innermost layer is called the intima. It's only a single cell layer thick and is composed of individual cells known as endothelial cells. These microscopic cells actually line the walls of all the blood vessels as well as the heart and perform many functions.[6]

One of these functions is to produce nitric oxide.[7] Nitric oxide is a gas (not to be confused with nitrous oxide—laughing gas). There's nothing funny about the vital nature of this task. It is needed to cause vasodilation of the smooth muscle cells surrounding the endothelial layer.[8] This allows for increased blood flow and a reduction in blood pressure. The importance of this function cannot be understated because hypertension (you know it as high blood pressure) is considered to be the leading risk factor—more than any other factor—in cardiovascular death and disability.[9] Hypertension is really only a symptom of cardiovascular disease, not a disease of its own. Nearly a third of the U.S. population is affected by hypertension making it an enormous problem.[10]

The next layer of the arterial wall is called the media, which is comprised mostly of vascular smooth muscle cells.[11] The ability of the vascular smooth muscle cells (VSMC) to undergo vasodilation and vasoconstriction (relaxing and contracting) to control blood pressure is one of its most important responsibilities. This process is highly dependent on nitric oxide production that I just talked about as a function of the first layer of cells.

Another important role of VSMC is the formation of new arteries and the remodeling of existing, injured arteries.[12] This happens more often in people who eat a rich Western diet composed of animal fats, saturated fats, and trans fats.[13] It just so happens that those French fries, chicken crispers, and beef cutlets are bad news for your coronary arteries. They damage the artery walls by flooding them full of cholesterol-laden plaques, and when the VSMC can't keep up with repairing the damage, the result is crushing chest pains and debilitating heart attacks.

The final and outermost layer of the artery is known as the adventitia. This layer consists of connective tissue, nerve cells, small blood vessels, and fat. It provides strength and integrity to the entire artery while preventing atherosclerotic lesions (plaques containing cholesterol and lipids) from eroding through the arterial wall and damaging adjacent tissues.[14]

It's important to understand these basic fundamental properties of the arterial wall in order to grasp the concept of how a clot develops. By doing so, it will help you understand the steps needed to prevent heart attacks and stroke. This next section explains the process.

Formation of an Atherosclerotic Plaque

Atherosclerotic plaques are the culprits behind every case of angina (chest pain), every heart attack, and the majority of strokes occurring today.[15] These plaques cause an enormous amount of damage to the walls of the arteries themselves, starting with the innermost endothelial cells.

The endothelial lining in its original healthy state is as smooth as glass, so blood flows freely throughout the entire cardiovascular system. There's literally no interference in blood flow if someone has no atherosclerotic plaques.

You can picture this by imagining water beading off the hood of a brand new car. The water slides right off the surface without obstruction, but over time this surface becomes nicked and scratched leaving a number of bumps and ridges behind. The water then has to find its way around these bumps and ridges before making its way to the ground. These nicks and scratches happen to our endothelial lining too. This causes injuries to the endothelial surface and leads to the formation of atherosclerotic plaques.

These initial injuries are primarily caused by elevated LDL "bad" cholesterol levels, high blood sugar, and high blood pressure, all of which are influenced greatly by our dietary choices.[16] Once the endothelial cells experience these injuries, nitric oxide production is reduced. This is due to the invasion of oxidized LDL cholesterol particles (LDL molecules previously attacked by free radicals), white blood cells and other harmful substances into the arterial walls. The result is a highly complex chain of events leading to further damage to the arteries.

A cascade of problems follows. First, the decrease in nitric oxide prevents the artery from dilating properly worsening one's blood pressure and putting more strain on the heart. This causes the heart to work harder. Second, the lack of nitric oxide causes the blood to become thicker and stickier. This is due to its inability to prevent platelet aggregation, inhibit leukocyte adhesion, and prevent the invasion of vascular smooth muscle cells into the growing plaque as it normally would.[17] In other words, particles in our blood start clumping together and sticking to the sides of our arteries. Not a healthy process for our blood vessels.

The next phase of the process involves macrophages. These are white blood cells called into action by our body to "gobble up" and dispose of the LDL particles now accumulating inside the artery wall. Instead of being able to "clean up" the cholesterol mess, these macrophages cause further damage by engulfing oxidized LDL molecules to form foam cells. Foam cells are basically oxidized LDL particles on steroids ready to wreak havoc on anything in their path. These foam cells release additional inflammatory markers along with harmful free radicals promoting more inflammation and oxidative damage to the surrounding cells and tissues.[18]

A progressive inflammatory response is now under way inside the arteries. This results in a vicious cycle of more white blood cells being recruited to the site of injury along with the enlistment of the vascular smooth muscle cells in the repair of the damaged artery wall. The accumulation of these extra white blood cells, smooth muscle cells, and foam cells now produces fatty streaks along the inside portion of the arteries and eventually leads to full-blown atherosclerotic plaques.

You might be surprised to learn that these fatty streaks start to develop early in life when we are still children. An article in the *American Journal of Clinical Nutrition* states that almost every North American child over the age of three has some degree of fatty streaks already forming inside their

NATURAL HISTORY OF ATHEROSCLEROSIS

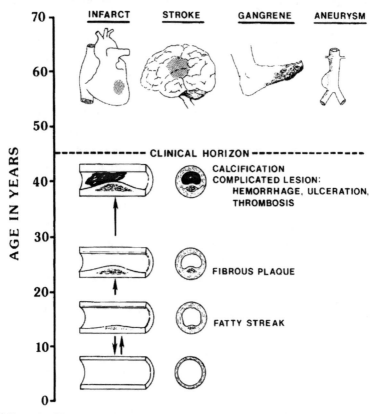

McGill et al., Chapter 2, Natural History of Human Atherosclerotic Lesions, pp 39–65, Atherosclerosis and its Origin, Eds. M. Sandler and G. Bourne, Academic Press, New York, 1963.

aorta—the largest artery in the body.[19] By the time these children reach puberty, more than half of them will have large accumulations of foam cells, extracellular lipids, and fat-laden smooth muscle cells inside portions of their artery walls.

As children reach young adulthood (in their late twenties) over a third will have well-developed, raised lesions, which will progress to advanced atherosclerotic plaques by the time they reach their forties, fifties, and sixties. The result is the out-of-control heart disease epidemic we are seeing today.

These dangerous plaques can rupture at any time, but normally do so in an unstable condition—still soft and tender with only a thin cap separating their lipid-rich core from the flow of blood inside the artery. In the event they rupture inside of a coronary artery, they block the flow of blood in the arteries surrounding the heart and a heart attack occurs.[20] If a rupture occurs inside an artery leading to the brain, blood flow is blocked to the brain and a stroke occurs.[21]

Well-established plaques typically do not cause heart attacks and strokes. Instead, these stable blockages are responsible for most of the cases of chronic chest pain or angina incurred by patients.[22] This warning sign should be taken seriously. The pain is caused by extensive hardening and calcification the arteries undergo causing major blockages in the coronary arteries. When someone talks about having an 80 percent or 90 percent blockage in one or more of their arteries, this is what they're referring to.

Conventional cardiologists are quick to resort to invasive procedures such as cardiac catheterizations or cardiac bypass surgeries when treating major blockages in the coronary arteries. It's not uncommon for people to hear of a close family member or friend going under the knife to "clean out" these blockages in an attempt to relieve their debilitating chest pain. During bypass surgery, this is accomplished by taking a blood vessel from another part of the body (leg, chest, or arm) and surgically attaching it to the other arteries around the heart, thereby bypassing the diseased or blocked artery.

However, there's a major downside to these operations. When these elective procedures are done and it's not an emergency, as opposed to using conservative noninvasive approaches such as diet and lifestyle interventions, the unblocking only succeeds in providing temporary relief at best with no real long-term benefit.

The *New England Journal of Medicine* concluded that cardiac catheterizations in patients with stable coronary artery disease do "not reduce the risk of death, myocardial infarction [commonly known as heart attacks], or other major cardiovascular events when added to optimal medical therapy."[23] Another article in the *American Journal of Cardiology* looked at two groups of patients with stable angina (bypass surgery patients versus medical management patients). Over a twenty-two-year period they found there was "no long-term survival benefit for high-risk patients assigned to bypass surgery" and the "trial provides strong evidence that initial bypass surgery did not improve survival for low-risk patients, and that it did not reduce the overall risk of myocardial infarction."[24]

Bypass surgeries have also been shown to carry some major risks, specifically when it comes to a person's brain health. It's been reported that 1 to 5 percent of patients suffer strokes during a bypass operation, another 10 to 28 percent suffer from delirium during the first week following surgery, and another 42 percent of patients will experience some form of cognitive dysfunction—most commonly memory loss—at the five-year mark after cardiac bypass surgery.[25] This means that a vast majority of nonemergency cardiac surgical interventions are performed without justification at the expense of a patient's physical, mental, emotional, and financial well-being.

It's sad that we've come to a point of such advances in modern medicine, but fail to use them in a responsible, effective manner when treating patients with cardiovascular disease. There has to be a better way. Fortunately, thanks to a distinguished physician who has already established his legendary status in the world of medicine, there is.

Trading Scalpels for Kitchen Utensils

In 1968 a bright young Army surgeon by the name of Caldwell Esselstyn Jr., MD, returned home from active duty after serving in Vietnam. Upon his return he landed a position as a general surgeon at the prestigious Cleveland Clinic—world renowned for its excellence in cardiovascular care. Dr. Esselstyn specialized in general surgery during most of his career but always had an interest in cardiovascular disease. This interest arose for a few reasons. First, it was the most fatal of any other chronic illness on the face of the planet. Second, heart disease had become personal for Dr. Esselstyn because it took away from him what no one can ever replace—his own father.

Over the years Dr. Esselstyn worked tirelessly to connect the dots between heart disease and nutrition as he buried himself in the medical literature. His passion for finding a cure was so intense that in 1985 he embarked on what is now known as the most successful scientific research study ever conducted on preventing and reversing heart disease. Dr. Esselstyn's work has since been published in numerous peer-reviewed scientific journals. He has also recounted much of his research in the book he wrote: *Prevent and Reverse Heart Disease*.

Dr. Esselstyn started his study on heart disease with a total of twenty-four participants. All study participants had advanced coronary artery disease (severe blockage), and many had failed previous cardiac bypass operations or angioplasties leaving them severely debilitated with crushing chest pain.[26] These patients had been referred to Dr. Esselstyn by fellow cardiologists after conventional medicine could do no more for them. They had literally been labeled as the walking dead by their former heart doctors. Dr. Esselstyn knew he could help.

He put these patients on a whole foods, plant-based lifestyle by eliminating all meat, dairy, eggs, and processed foods from their diet. He encouraged them to eat as much as they wanted of four main food groups—fruits, vegetables, whole grains, and legumes. No rigorous exercise program was required, but it was also not discouraged if subjects wanted to exercise on their own.

Cholesterol-lowering medications were used, but only at the lowest possible dose and *only* in those who couldn't achieve a total cholesterol of less than 150 mg/dl following Dr. Esselstyn's dietary program. (A total cholesterol of less than 150 mg/dl had been chosen as the target goal because it had been proven in the past to eliminate all cases of coronary heart disease.)[27]

Six patients failed to remain compliant with Dr. Esselstyn's program during the first twelve to eighteen months. They were released from the study back to their regular doctors. Over a decade later these same individuals experienced a total of thirteen new cardiac events (such as heart attacks or chest pain).[28] The remaining eighteen patients all stayed compliant with the program for the first five years, and only one patient became noncompliant after the five-year point. At the five-year mark, eleven patients underwent an angiography (imaging, like an x-ray) to determine the disease status of their blood vessels.

The results were unexpected. All the patients had completely halted their heart disease. All of them! A 100 percent success rate was unheard of when it came to treating heart disease up until then. The outcome was in most clinicians' minds a medical miracle.

In addition, eight of the remaining eleven patients had actually *reversed* their disease from the original starting point. Their coronary plaques had essentially diminished from their beginning level. These kinds of results had never before been seen in any drug trial or any other medical trial in human history. Dr. Esselstyn had truly achieved greatness with his revolutionary and groundbreaking work.

The most compelling evidence of all that Dr. Esselstyn's eating style works can be found in looking at the number of cardiac events that occurred in compliant patients before and after the study began. Before starting the program a total of forty-nine cardiac events during the previous eight years had occurred in the compliant group of patients. After starting the study, and for the next twelve years, there wasn't a single new cardiac event (no heart attack, no stroke, no angina) in these same patients. It's as if their heart disease had literally been wiped completely off their medical record. Nobody had ever been able to accomplish such remarkable results before. This outcome speaks volumes for how important proper nutrition and a plant-based lifestyle can be when tackling the number one killer—cardiovascular disease.

So Why Not Just Take Statins?

Many may wonder why not just pop a statin pill and medicate your problems away? That's a fair question, requiring a thoughtful answer.

While a select few may benefit from taking statin drugs, which are used to lower cholesterol levels with such popular names as Crestor and Lipitor, the vast majority of heart disease patients do not benefit.[29] A look at the evidence for statin use in primary prevention (individuals who *have never* suffered a cardiovascular event before) versus secondary prevention (individuals who *have suffered* a previous cardiovascular event) shows why. The following data are from theNNT Reviews (thennt.com).

As a bit of background information, theNNT (Numbers Needed to Treat) is a group of physicians dedicated to providing both medical professionals and the general public with unbiased, independent reviews of the scientific literature on various diseases and their treatments. theNNT strictly prohibits financial contributions of any kind from industry sources—pharmaceutical, medical device, or insurance companies. They truly offer fair reviews of the scientific and medical literature in hopes of putting patient-centered outcomes first instead of corporate interests.

While examining the literature for statin use in primary prevention efforts for cardiovascular disease, theNNT's overall conclusions found "no benefits" after five years of therapy.[30] The following is a detailed description of these findings:

- 98% saw no benefits from taking statins
- 0% were helped in terms of lives saved
- 1.6% were helped by preventing a heart attack (1 in 60)
- 0.4% were helped by preventing a stroke (1 in 268)
- 2% were harmed by developing diabetes (1 in 50)
- 10% were harmed by muscle damage (1 in 10)

For statin use in secondary prevention theNNT's overall conclusions found that "benefits outweigh harms" after five years of therapy.[31] Here is the detailed description of their findings:

- 96% saw no benefits from taking statins
- 1.2% were helped in terms of lives saved (1 in 83)

- 2.6% were helped by preventing a repeat nonfatal heart attack (1 in 39)
- 0.8% were helped by preventing a stroke (1 in 125)
- 2% were harmed by developing diabetes (1 in 50)
- 10% were harmed by muscle damage (1 in 10)

Another comprehensive review analyzing multiple studies on statin use was published in 2013 by two vascular surgeons in Europe in the *Journal of Endocrine and Metabolic Diseases*.[32] These physicians declared no financial conflicts of interest with any industry ties and came to the same conclusions as theNNT—statin drugs showed a clear benefit in secondary, but not primary, prevention efforts in cardiovascular disease.

The authors found several disconcerting adverse effects in healthy adults who took statin drugs for primary prevention. These adverse effects include an increased risk of diabetes, cataract formation, and erectile dysfunction in the young; increased incidence of coronary artery calcifications (calcium deposits in the arteries) in type 2 diabetics and women; and cancer and neurodegenerative disorders in the elderly.

They also stated in their review that they "discovered that for every 10,000 people taking a statin, there were 307 extra patients with cataracts, 23 additional patients with acute kidney failure and 74 extra patients with liver dysfunction. Furthermore, statin therapy increased muscle fatigability by 30% with 11.3% incidence of rhabdomyolysis at high doses." Rhabdomyolysis is a severe muscle condition where the breakdown and destruction of muscle fiber occurs causing muscle pain and weakness.

After reviewing the data on statin therapy, it is evident that anyone considering taking these medications examine them with due diligence. Have a thoughtful discussion on both the benefits and risks with your doctor. An informed decision can then be made, with careful deliberation on the known facts, as to whether or not you choose to use these medications.

Other Important Points in the Battle Against Heart Disease

To wrap up the discussion on heart disease, a few additional points on nutrition and heart health are in order. These relate to cardiac arrhythmias.

Heart arrhythmias happen when the electrical impulses responsible for coordinating a regular heart rhythm do not fire correctly. The result is irregular heartbeats, abnormally slow heartbeats, or unusually fast heartbeats. Individuals experiencing this may complain of a fluttering or racing heart. Most of the time heart arrhythmias are relatively harmless, but sometimes they can become severe or even life threatening, leading to sudden cardiac death.

Common arrhythmias include atrial fibrillation, ventricular tachycardia, and ventricular fibrillation—the terms you hear on TV doctor shows. Conventional therapy normally consists of an array of prescription drugs including beta blockers, calcium channel blockers, amiodarone, digoxin, and other medications to treat these conditions. Many times patients will be put on multiple drugs at the same time to try to control their arrhythmias. Although these approaches are appropriate after an arrhythmia develops, adopting a plant-based lifestyle can dramatically reduce your risk of experiencing an arrhythmia in the first place.

Cardiac arrhythmias, and more specifically atrial fibrillation, have been linked to the consumption of the high-fat Western diet.[33] This is thought to be due to both atherosclerotic plaque formation along with an excessive amount of omega-6 fatty acids in the diet.[34] Omega-6 fatty acids are pro-inflammatory and can lead to negative health consequences when consumed in large amounts.

Omega-6 fatty acids are found in high quantities in foods such as vegetable oils (olive oil included), meat, dairy, and eggs. In contrast, foods containing high amounts of heart-healthy omega-3 fatty acids have been shown to protect and prevent against cardiac arrhythmias.[35] These foods include flaxseeds, chia seeds, and dark leafy greens among other plant-based foods.

The omega-3 fatty acid commonly found in plant-based foods is known as alpha-linolenic acid (ALA). The omega-3 fatty acids commonly found in fish are known as eicosapentaenoic acid (EPA) and docosahexaenoic acid (DHA). EPA and DHA are the forms of omega-3 utilized by the body to prevent a number of chronic diseases, including heart disease. When we consume ALA from plants, it is converted to EPA and DHA by the body.[36]

You would think that consuming fish would be the best way to obtain heart-healthy omega-3, but this is not the case. A study published in 2012 looked at omega-3 consumption from fish and the risk of sudden cardiac death (SCD).[37] SCD is often preceded by cardiac arrhythmias. Researchers found that high exposures to toxic levels of mercury in the fish significantly reduced the benefits of their omega-3 fatty acid composition and the resulting incidences of SCD.

In contrast, obtaining omega-3 fatty acids from plant-based sources carries no risk of heavy metal intoxication and still provides the much needed protection from SCD. A study in the journal *Circulation* looked at 76,763 women in the Nurses' Health Study and their subsequent intake of ALA.[38] Researchers found that as ALA consumption from plant foods increased, the women's risk of SCD decreased. This benefit persisted even after controlling for the intake of other dietary fats, including fish consumption.

Obtaining omega-3 from plant-based sources such as dark leafy greens or various seeds high in ALA content is the safest way to get the heart-healthy benefits they supply to the cardiovascular system.

Role of Arginine in Heart Health

L-arginine, a common amino acid, plays a critical role in maintaining a healthy cardiovascular system. It does so by acting as a precursor for the production of nitric oxide.[39] By combining with oxygen—during an enzymatic reaction—L-arginine is subsequently converted to nitric oxide, which as you already know is vital to maintaining a healthy endothelial lining in the arteries. Without arginine there would be no nitric oxide, and without nitric oxide your cardiovascular system would be in total disarray.

The best sources of arginine are heart-healthy plant foods. These include legumes, nuts and seeds, potatoes (including sweet potatoes), fruit, and green and yellow vegetables.[40] All of these foods should serve as a strong foundation to a heart-healthy lifestyle. By adopting this style of eating, you can free yourself of the worries of future heart attacks and strokes regardless of your family history. This should be a priority for anyone wishing to avoid the world's deadliest serial killer.

Winning the Battle Against Type 2 Diabetes

"It looks to me to be obvious that the whole world cannot eat an American diet."

—JERRY BROWN

Each morning millions of Americans wake up to the rays of the sun peeking through their windows, a fresh pot of coffee brewing in the kitchen, and a hearty breakfast of bacon, eggs, and pancakes awaiting them. Little do they know that over time these foods will eventually lead to one of the most debilitating illnesses one could ever suffer.

Diabetes is now a formidable player in the world of chronic diseases. It's one of the fastest growing diseases affecting advanced nations. Why? Because of the rising rate of obesity. Rich foods, a sedentary lifestyle, and a symptom-based approach to treating diabetes is fueling this epidemic.

According to 2010 data from the Centers for Disease Control and Prevention (CDC), a little more than one of every ten adults (11.3%) is currently diagnosed with diabetes in the United States, 25.6 million people in total.[1] Type 2 diabetes accounts for 90 to 95 percent of all diagnosed cases. Another 79 million people have prediabetes, a condition that increases the risk of developing type 2 diabetes, heart disease, and stroke.

Together these two conditions result in a total of 104.6 million people (one of every three adults) living with these illnesses in the U.S. These conditions can lead to devastating health effects down the road including high blood pressure, heart disease, kidney failure, blindness, hearing loss, peripheral neuropathy, skin infections, skin ulcers, impotence, depression, peripheral arterial disease, stroke, limb amputations, and even premature death.

Thankfully, there are a number of things that can be done in order to prevent or even reverse type 2 diabetes. But first, an understanding of the disease process itself is critical.

An Overview of Type 2 Diabetes

The scientific world has provided us with an enormous amount of useful information in understanding how type 2 diabetes develops in the human body. While we will always continue to learn more about this disease, the latest research has pointed to three major factors playing a significant role in the development of type 2 diabetes—insulin resistance, excess fat in the muscle cells, and the body's inability to adequately regulate energy metabolism.

Insulin Resistance

Insulin resistance is the first of these factors and is usually the *only* factor talked about whenever the word *diabetes* comes up in conversation. You hear about insulin resistance when talking to friends and family. You also hear about it at the doctor's office.

Insulin resistance occurs when a person's fat, muscle, and liver cells do not respond appropriately to the actions of insulin, which in turn leads to elevated blood glucose levels. In other words, your body does not properly use insulin the way it was designed to.

Insulin and Fat Cells. Under normal circumstances when the body is in a fasting state, adipose tissue (body fat) will undergo a process called lipolysis to provide the body with energy. Lipolysis occurs when fat is broken down into free fatty acids (FFA). These FFAs are then released into the blood supply to be used as energy.[2] However, when you eat, there is an outpouring of insulin (via the pancreas) that suppresses this process of lipolysis preventing the release of FFAs into the blood supply.

This makes perfect sense if you think about it because the body doesn't need to use its own fat stores for energy while eating. It can obtain all the energy needed from the foods being consumed at that very moment.

Things change in the case of obese individuals. For them, insulin resistance often prevents the suppression of lipolysis during the fed state, resulting in FFAs—those tiny individual fat particles—being released into the blood supply.[3] Since the blood supply is now overloaded with fat, it leads to the redistribution of these extra fat particles to nonadipose tissues such as skeletal muscle cells and liver cells causing further progression of type 2 diabetes.[4]

Insulin and Muscle Cells. After you eat, insulin in the bloodstream finds its way to an insulin receptor on the outer surface of muscle cells and attaches itself there. If everything goes as planned, a cascade of signaling events begins to unfold. A glucose transporter called GLUT4 (also sitting on the outer membrane of the muscle cell) is activated by insulin's attachment to an insulin receptor.[5] GLUT4 is responsible for transporting glucose from the bloodstream into the muscle cell in order for it to be used as energy.[6] Essentially, GLUT4 is the "doorway" for glucose to enter the muscle cell.

Insulin resistance significantly decreases this whole process, which is a major concern because skeletal muscle is responsible for 70 to 90 percent of glucose disposal after consuming a meal. If this chain of events isn't working properly, then glucose stays in the bloodstream instead of being shuffled through the "doorways" of the muscle cells. Consequently, an individual's blood sugar has only one way to go ... UP!

Insulin and Liver Cells. In the liver, insulin plays two major roles. First, after you eat a meal, insulin signals the liver to store extra glucose in the form of glycogen.[7] Second, when you are eating a meal, insulin directs the liver to stop the breakdown of already stored glycogen since these extra sources of glucose (that is, energy) are not needed at that time.

Insulin resistance disrupts these two processes leading to extra glucose being dumped into the bloodstream. This results in higher blood glucose levels and advances the disease process itself.

Increased Intramyocellular Lipids (IMCL)

Intramyocellular lipids (IMCL) are little particles of fat (in other words, free fatty acids or FFAs) located inside muscle cells. You may have never heard about IMCLs. Most people haven't. But the topic of IMCLs is extremely important when discussing the development of diabetes because *it is the main culprit behind insulin resistance.* However, this process is often ignored, unknowingly in most cases, by the physicians, dietitians, pharmacists, and other healthcare professionals treating diabetes.

Neal Barnard, MD, along with a handful of other medical doctors, is an exception to this rule. He has brought much of this research to light, leading to a better understanding of the root cause of type 2 diabetes. If you don't understand the role of IMCLs in type 2 diabetes, then you'll never defeat this disease.

All muscle cells have a small number of IMCLs inside them. These fat particles are used for periods of time when the body doesn't have enough glucose to meet its energy demands, such as between meals. However, a high number of IMCLs in muscle cells is detrimental and is linked in obese individuals to higher rates of insulin resistance.[8] Type 2 diabetics, who are often overweight or obese, have an excess supply of IMCLs in their muscle cells.

An overabundance of IMCLs causes serious problems in overweight people due to the production of lipid metabolites, namely diacylglycerol (DAG) and ceramide, which interfere with insulin signaling.[9,10] DAG and ceramide impede the insulin-signaling cascade that allows GLUT4 to transport glucose from the bloodstream into the muscle cells so that it can be used for energy.[11] Let me simplify: Extra fat in the diet ends up short circuiting the "doorways" of the muscle cells preventing glucose from getting through the door. Therefore, glucose stays in the bloodstream and blood sugar levels rise. This is insulin resistance in action. Needless to say, those extra particles of fat (IMCLs) are a big reason why insulin resistance develops in the first place.

An excess of these IMCL metabolites provides a double whammy for at-risk individuals by activating a number of substances leading to an inflammatory response in the body.[12] This inflammatory response has been shown to be another cause of insulin resistance in obese and type 2 diabetic patients.

If the topic of IMCLs were explained in a way that medical professionals and patients better understood, then their significance could be emphasized in reducing or eliminating this horrible disease. Drugs will never be able to medicate away the extra fat consumed in the Western diet. Pharmaceutical companies are, therefore, only offering a Band-Aid by treating type 2 diabetes with medications.

Reduction in PGC-1α

Most people have never heard of peroxisome proliferator-activated receptor gamma coactivator 1-alpha (PGC-1α). It certainly is a mouthful!

PGC-1α also plays an important role in the development of type 2 diabetes. It is responsible for regulating energy metabolism. It acts as a major activator of mitochondrial biogenesis.[13] Mitochondrial biogenesis is the formation of new mitochondria within the body's cells. This is important especially when referring to muscle cells because mitochondria act like little power plants.[14] Their job is to produce the energy needed for muscle cells to carry out their daily functions.

If mitochondria are considered the power plants of these cells, then PGC-1α would be considered one of the chief engineers in charge of building these power plants. This is a big responsibility indeed, but why is this important?

Because mitochondria love glucose. Glucose is the key ingredient used by mitochondria to make energy. It's their primary source of fuel. In obesity and type 2 diabetes there is a reduced expression of PGC-1α, which reduces the body's ability to utilize available glucose.[15,16] In other words, overweight and diabetic individuals have a harder time using the body's best source of fuel—glucose. It should make sense why those with extra body weight and diabetes are so exhausted all the time. Fewer chief engineers (PGC-1α) equal fewer power plants (mitochondria), which means less energy being produced. It's as simple as that.

Pills to the Rescue? How about Insulin?

If you have type 2 diabetes or know someone with type 2 diabetes, then the typical course of treatment goes like this:

- Go to the doctor. Type 2 diabetes diagnosed.
- Diet and exercise are prescribed.
- Return in three to six months. Diet and exercise didn't work.
- Anti-diabetic pills are prescribed.
- Anti-diabetic pills lose effectiveness over the course of months to years.
- Insulin is added to antidiabetic pill regimen.
- Type 2 diabetes progresses despite the use of antidiabetic pills and insulin. Serious complications and eventually premature death follow.

You can't blame your doctor for this scenario. Like pharmacists, well-meaning physicians are only doing what they were taught in school—medicate the disease. By medicating the disease it is hoped to manage blood sugar levels more appropriately over time leading to less microvascular complications (kidney, eye, and nerve damage) and macrovascular complications (strokes, heart disease, peripheral vascular disease, and amputations).[17]

The gold standard for measuring the success of a drug is its ability to reduce a blood test known as hemoglobin A1C (you hear it called *ay-one-see*). The A1C is a good indicator of average blood sugar levels over a two- to three-month period. It gives the clinician and patient a better overall picture of how controlled (or uncontrolled) a person's diabetes is.

The A1C level of nondiabetics is usually less than 5.7 percent. Prediabetic people have an A1C level between 5.7 and 6.4. Diabetic patients have an A1C level of 6.5 or higher. Many out-of-control diabetics will have A1C levels of 8, 9, or even 10 or higher. Remember, using medications to treat diabetes and target certain A1C ranges only serves to *manage* the disease. It does not get rid of it. While this strategy can reduce complications in some cases, individuals remain diabetic using this approach. Patients also have to mitigate the side effects of the medications they're using. Some of these can be serious too.

The following is a look at popular antidiabetic medications and their potential A1C reduction, and possible common or serious side effects:[18-20]

(1) Biguanides (metformin)
A1C reduction: 1.0–2.0%
Possible side effects: Nausea, diarrhea, abdominal pain, decreased appetite. Considered safest of all antidiabetic medications. May even mitigate some of the side effects of other antidiabetic drugs when used in combination therapy.

(2) Sulfonylureas (glyburide, glimepiride, are examples)
A1C reduction: 1.0–2.0%
Possible side effects: Severe low blood sugar (hypoglycemia) accompanied by coma or seizures, weight gain.

(3) Thiazolidinediones (Actos, Avandia)
A1C reduction: 0.5–1.4%
Possible side effects: Fluid retention, weight gain, increased risk of congestive heart failure (CHF), bone fractures, three- to six-fold increased risk of macular edema (retina damage and blindness). Avandia carries a 30%–40% increased risk of heart attacks.

(4) Glucagon-like peptide-1 receptor agonists (Byetta, Victoza)
A1C reduction: 0.5–1.0%
Possible side effects: Nausea, vomiting, severe pancreatitis. Byetta

may cause acute kidney damage/failure. Victoza caused thyroid cancer in animal studies and carries an FDA warning about possible thyroid tumors developing. Long-term safety of these agents has not been established.

(5) Dipeptidyl Peptidase-4 Inhibitors (Januvia, Tradjenta, Onglyza)
A1C reduction: 0.5–0.8%
Possible side effects: Nausea, diarrhea, abdominal pain, increased incidence of infections, severe pancreatitis. Long-term safety of these agents has not been established.

(6) Insulin (Regular, NPH, Lispro, Lantus, Levemir, and others)
A1C reduction: 1.5–3.5%
Possible side effects: Severe hypoglycemia, weight gain. Insulin therapy was associated with worse outcomes for cardiovascular events, stroke, cancer, neuropathy, eye complications, kidney disease, and overall incidence of death compared to diabetics treated with only metformin.

Hope in the Form of Lifestyle Medicine

Conventional medicine practitioners approach type 2 diabetes with less-than-adequate advice on nutrition and exercise. Instead, they place a large emphasis on pills, pills, and more pills. Throw in a little insulin when the pills stop working and you have yourself the typical type 2 diabetic a handful of years after he or she has been diagnosed—overmedicated and feeling miserable.

There's a reason for this. Approaching type 2 diabetes on the back end with medications attempts only to put a Band-Aid on the problem instead of addressing the root cause of the disease. Unlike antibiotics that are taken to cure infections, the medications taken for diabetes only serve as a prelude for further complications and further progression of this disease. They do nothing to cure it.

It's hard to win the war on diabetes when the only topic of conversation focuses on insulin resistance. By doing so, we are ignoring the more pressing subjects of increased IMCLs and decreased mitochondrial biogenesis. This is why mainstream medicine flourishes while doing nothing to dramatically reduce or eliminate this horrific disease.

A shift in our nation's approach to this disease is critically needed from both the healthcare profession and the public. A new emphasis on lifestyle medicine must be implemented. Primary focus should be on nutritional excellence if we are to defeat this disease once and for all.

To get to the root cause of type 2 diabetes, it's absolutely essential to remove the offending agents responsible for causing the imbalances learned about in the beginning of this chapter. These offending agents include animal-based and processed foods, as well as a sedentary lifestyle.

Whole Foods Restore Health

Eating whole, plant-based foods is exactly what one should strive to do to beat type 2 diabetes. Type 2 diabetes can be completely reversed by adopting a plant-based lifestyle consisting of the following foods:

- Vegetables
- Fruits
- Legumes (beans, lentils, and peas, for example)
- Whole grains
- Nuts/seeds (optional)

Keep in mind that it's just as important to stay away from animal-based foods (meat, dairy, and eggs) as well as their equally harmful counterparts of processed foods. These items tend to be much higher in fat, especially trans and saturated fat, which are leading risk factors in the development of type 2 diabetes.

Even a diet high in fish, filled with omega-3 fatty acids, has been shown to increase the risk of type 2 diabetes by up to 46 percent in some cases.[21] These data come from the Women's Health Study that followed 36,328 women over a sixteen-year period. This same study showed that omega-3 fatty acid intake from plant-based sources did not have the same risk of developing type 2 diabetes.

> **Even a diet high in fish, filled with omega-3 fatty acids, has been shown to increase the risk of type 2 diabetes by up to 46 percent.**

Oils are another food item that needs to be avoided in order to give yourself the best chance of reversing type 2 diabetes. All oils (including olive, canola, and coconut oil) are processed foods and contain 100 percent of their calories from fat. Many studies have indicated that substituting saturated fats (found in items such as meat and dairy) with unsaturated fats (found in vegetable oils) does lead to lower rates of type 2 diabetes.[22] However, while a reduction in diabetes is seen in these cases, it is not the same as reversing the disease. It's the equivalent of squirting only a small amount of gasoline onto a fire instead of dumping a five-gallon bucket of gasoline onto it. Both actions continue to feed the fire. Instead, the best choice is to stop fueling the fire in the first place. Stay away from these highly processed forms of pure fat.

The unsaturated fatty acids found in oils and other foods do not promote reversal of diabetes and only have the potential to cause harm to beta cells in the pancreas. Beta cells are responsible for producing insulin. This is important since insulin is needed by the body to properly metabolize glucose. According to research published in 2009 analyzing beta cell function and fat intake, "A vast excess of almost any fatty acid is likely to be detrimental under some circumstances, irrespective of its chain length or double bond configuration."[23] This is the same as saying both saturated and unsaturated fatty acids can be damaging to your health. Both play a role in worsening type 2 diabetes.

Adopt a Whole Foods, Plant-Based Eating Style

A review of fourteen randomized controlled clinical trials over a ten-year period highlighted the importance of adopting a low-fat, plant-based eating style compared to other commonly accepted diets when treating type 2 diabetes.[24] Individuals adopting a plant-based lifestyle saw a marked increase in insulin sensitivity and glucose metabolism compared to other dieters. They also experienced greater improvements in their cholesterol levels, body weight, and A1C levels than other dieters.

I've created a table on the next page comparing two different dinner meals recommended for diabetics. One meal is from the Physicians Committee for Responsible Medicine (PCRM) and the other by the American Diabetes Association (ADA).[25,26] PCRM's plant-based meal is much healthier and has a lower fat content—and includes brownies. PCRM has been using this approach to help patients reverse type 2 diabetes for several years. Note the dramatic difference in number of calories and percentage of the meal from fat. That's my point.

In contrast, the ADA's meal is typical of most common diets where little, if any, change has been made in comparison with the status quo. Both the ADA's diet, other popular diets, and even the Standard American Diet (SAD) contain approximately 20 to 35 percent of their calories from fat. None of these diets have ever produced consistent results in reversing type 2 diabetes.

Unfortunately, the general public and healthcare professionals look to the ADA for guidance when treating type 2 diabetes. Therefore, the advice you may be getting from your doctor or dietitian is promoting the progression of diabetes instead of helping you reverse it.

PCRM's Plant-Based Dinner			ADA's Diabetic Dinner		
Food Item	Calories	% Calories from fat	Food Item	Calories	% Calories from fat
Aztec salad	158	6.5	Arugula and watercress salad (with olive oil dressing)	80	70
Mexican skillet pie	192	13.6	Mini Greek chicken kabobs	60	41.7
Quick confetti rice	94	7.1	Cheese and rice stuffed peppers	283	9.5
Brownies	50	6.2	Cherry and toasted almond pie	232	37.1
Total	494	9.3	Total	655	29.6

The Importance of Getting Your Exercise

While nutrition serves as the foundation for defeating type 2 diabetes, regular exercise also plays an important role. At least three hours a week of moderate exercise (such as walking, swimming, or biking) should be your goal. These three hours can be broken up into shorter segments of ten to thirty minutes each or whatever works best for you.

Exercise is so important in improving diabetes for a number of reasons including the following:

- The combination of weight loss and exercise has been shown to decrease insulin resistance in patients.[27]
- Exercise has been shown to increase the number of mitochondria in cells thereby increasing glucose metabolism and reducing insulin

resistance leading to improved A1C and fasting blood glucose levels in type 2 diabetic patients.[28] This is accomplished by increasing the amount of PGC-1α content in skeletal muscle.[29]

- An increase in PGC-1α expression due to regular exercise also helps improve the efficiency of certain types of muscle fibers so they produce more energy by using up the available glucose supply in the blood.[30]

All of this comes back to doing the basics right—eating healthy and exercising regularly. Dr. Neal Barnard (President of PCRM) has been advocating for these simple approaches for years and has had tremendous success in treating his patients. His book, *Dr. Neal Barnard's Program for Reversing Diabetes*, outlines how this approach has reversed this deadly disease in thousands of patients over the past few decades. It's a must read for anyone wishing to take back control of their own health.

My Story (written by Cherise Scally)

My name is Cherise Scally, and I suffered from type 2 diabetes for eleven years and nine months before reversing it with a plant-based, raw foods diet and exercise. It all started when I remarried and tried to have another child. We lost our first child to medical complications unrelated to diabetes. During my third pregnancy I developed this dreadful disease that never went away. We lost our second daughter due to complications of diabetes at twenty-six weeks.

There was no history of diabetes on either side of our family except for my father who had been diagnosed around the time we found out I was pregnant with our second child. After suffering the loss of our second child, we were able to successfully bring home our miracle child two years later. Our son had his share of problems due to my disease. He was born with a hole in his heart a month early and lived the first month of his life in the NICU.

During the time from being diagnosed and reversing my diabetes, not one of my many doctors ever told me I could be free of this disease. I was told routinely that I would have to learn how to live with this disease and hope to minimize the damage it would cause me. I was never told that the treatment of my disease would ensure that I stayed ill the rest of my life. The treatment for diabetes is to manage the symptoms by pills and insulin to the detriment of the diabetic. Both treatments cause weight gain for a patient who is already in most cases overweight, which in turn causes more pills and insulin to be prescribed to control blood sugar. It is a vicious, painful, and devastating way to live.

One day I decided I was tired of being sick and there had to be a way to beat this. That is when I began my journey to wellness and just recently wrote a book about it: *A Personal Journey to Reverse Type 2 Diabetes.* In the pages of my book you will follow me from the loss of our first child, second child, birth of our son and my quest to find the answer to be free of diabetes. I did what I was told was not possible, I reversed diabetes and have been diabetes free for eight months now.

Thankfully I have reversed any and all damage the disease and treatment caused me. Type 2 diabetes regardless of how you get it can be reversed not by modern medicine but by food. This is a fundamental truth that you won't hear from most of the medical profession. I was not given this life-saving information from anyone in the medical field; for me it came from a friend who lives a plant-based lifestyle. I am grateful for her sharing the life-saving principles of this way of life. Now this is my way of life and I am on a new journey to share this information with others so that they can find their way to a life without disease.

5

A Cancer-Free Life—
Is It Possible?

"Cancer is not a death sentence, but rather it is a life sentence; it pushes one to live."

—MARCIA SMITH

More people fear cancer than any other disease in the world. The Harvard School of Public Health recently revealed this fact when between 40 and 49 percent of respondents admitted this fear in a survey.[1] Why is it we fear cancer so much? After all, it causes only half as many deaths worldwide as cardiovascular disease.[2] In addition, a third of all cancers are preventable simply by avoiding excessive alcohol consumption and by abstaining from smoking.[3] So why is it that people stop dead in their tracks when they hear the word *cancer*?

The reason may very well be the pain and suffering that's anticipated while undergoing the aggressive treatments of surgery, chemotherapy, and radiation. Constant pain, sleepless nights, lack of appetite, nausea/vomiting, severe weakness, and even the loss of hair are just a few of the unpleasant side effects that most people think of with cancer treatment. Sometimes the thought of death itself is more comforting than these horrific side effects.

To make matters worse, there's never a guarantee that these treatments or any other form of treatment will even work when all is said and done. In the end death may be inevitable no matter what one does to avoid it. It's this nightmare scenario that makes people cringe at the very mention of cancer.

Hope is something people try to hold on to though. It's a big reason why so many forge ahead refusing to give up on this new predicament they find themselves in. As long as there's a chance, people will do anything to defeat cancer. I hope that by reading this chapter your mind will be opened to a whole new line of treatment and prevention options for cancer that you may never have even heard of or thought possible before.

Optimum nutrition is at the heart of what's discussed in this chapter. Eating foods that fight cancer and avoiding foods that promote the growth of existing tumors should be of prime concern in any cancer patient's plan of attack. Nutritional excellence can not only complement conventional treatments but also force some forms of cancer to go into remission. The amazing power of a whole foods, plant-based lifestyle accomplishes this in a number of different ways as you will soon find out.

The Hidden Dangers of Animal Protein

One of the most profound links between nutrition and cancer involves animal-based proteins. Casein, an animal protein found in dairy products, is arguably considered one of the most powerful cancer promoters ever studied in scientific research.

Casein makes up approximately 80 percent of all protein in cow's milk with the remaining portion consisting of whey protein.[4] The link between casein and cancer progression was first uncovered in the 1960s by Indian research scientists.[5] They conducted animal experiments where rats were injected with aflatoxin—a powerful known and potent carcinogen (causes cancer). The rats were then given varying amounts of dietary protein (casein). One group received 5 percent of their total calories from protein, and the other received 20 percent.

The group that received 20 percent protein all developed liver cancer and eventually died from the disease. The group that received 5 percent protein fared much better. Not a single case of cancer was seen in this group. Not one case! This shocking discovery stirred a lot of controversy throughout the scientific community.

Like many of us, researchers and scientists all grew up assuming that animal protein was superior to plant protein since it served as a complete source of all the essential amino acids. No one would have ever thought of questioning this fact. It was commonly accepted that milk was good for you, along with all other dairy products coming from the cow's udder. With this study the widely accepted notion of dairy products serving as a health food was being called out and in a rather shocking way.

Many experts refused to believe these data. Animal proteins couldn't possibly act as potent cancer promoters, they thought. Skepticism was rampant, and such was the case when renowned nutritional research scientist Dr. T. Colin Campbell reviewed these results. Dr. Campbell was especially skeptical since he had grown up on a dairy farm. To him milk was the ultimate health food promoting the growth of strong, healthy bones needed to put in a hard day's work on the farm. He wasn't about to brush these reports under the rug, though, like many other experts had. Instead, he proceeded to follow up with his own studies to confirm the validity, or lack thereof, of the original research.

What followed would change the course of nutritional science forever. Dr. Campbell confirmed the link between liver cancer and animal protein intake just like his Indian predecessors.[6] In subsequent experiments he was able to *turn on* and *turn off* cancer growth simply by altering the amount of protein given to rats. Dr. Campbell found that when animal protein intake rose above 10 percent of total calories, cancer growth was turned on and tumor progression ensued.[7] When fewer than 10 percent of calories were consumed as animal protein, cancer was turned off. It was as easy as turning on or off a light switch.

This was truly an amazing discovery in the scientific world. The question that remained now was whether this association between cancer and protein consumption just involved animal-based proteins or did plant-based proteins also pose a concern?

Dr. Campbell wanted to find this out so he set out to test two commonly consumed proteins derived from plants—wheat and soy. What he found was just as shocking as the previous data.

The consumption of these proteins *did not* result in cancer growth like the casein did.[8,9] The same study design as with animal-based protein was put in place. Two groups of rats received doses of the potent carcinogen aflatoxin and then were fed varying amounts of wheat and soy proteins (5% vs. 20%). All animals studied remained in perfect health and actually thrived on the plant-based proteins. Even when 20 percent of calories were consumed from these plant-based proteins, there was absolutely no sign of cancer in any of the animals being studied.

It had now become clear to Dr. Campbell and the rest of the research community that while potent carcinogens such as aflatoxin were responsible for the initiation of cancer, the type and amount of protein consumed in one's diet played a significant role in the progression of cancer. Animal-based protein, such as casein, had now been proven to be a lethal promoter of our most dreaded disease when consumed in large amounts.

Human Nutritional Studies and Cancer

Studies confirming dairy protein and cancer risk in laboratory animals are one thing but what about humans? Do all animal-based proteins and the fats that accompany them increase one's risk of cancer or does this just apply to laboratory rats?

One thing is certain. This continues to be a heated topic among many in our culture creating some very divisive views. While research still needs to be done to hammer out all the details, a growing body of evidence favors consuming less animal foods and more plant foods to prevent and even treat various cancers.

Dairy and Cancer

When we look specifically at the link between dairy and cancer, two compelling studies echo a larger body of evidence that dairy consumption and cancer go hand in hand within the human population:

- **The Boyd Orr Cohort Study.** Over 4,000 people were followed for a period of sixty-five years in this study making it one of the longest studies ever conducted on dairy consumption and cancer risk. Researchers concluded that high childhood total dairy intake was associated with an increased risk of developing colorectal cancer in adulthood.[10] This risk was almost threefold higher for those consuming the most dairy and was independent of childhood meat, fruit, and vegetable intakes or socioeconomic status.
- **Swedish Based Study on Dairy/Calcium Intake and Prostate Cancer.** This study showed that high consumption of dairy products significantly increased the chances of men developing prostate cancer.[11] Even after adjusting for age, family history of prostate cancer, total average caloric intake, and smoking, there was still a 50 percent increased risk of prostate cancer in men consuming high amounts of dairy products.

The increased risk of these two particular cancers should sound alarm bells if it hasn't already for you because of the widespread prevalence of these two forms of cancer. According to the American Cancer Society, the *number one* projected cancer in 2013 in terms of newly diagnosed cases is prostate cancer with an estimated 238,590 cases.[12] Prostate cancer topped both breast and lung cancer, which came in second and third, respectively. Colorectal cancer wasn't too far behind with an estimated 142,820 new cases expected to be diagnosed in 2013. Avoiding dairy products and finding alternate substitutes may just be the next best thing you could do to reduce your risk of these common cancers.

Meat Consumption and Cancer

What about meat consumption? Is the risk of cancer just as high for the most prized centerpiece of the majority of American meals? The answer is yes!

It turns out that eating meat, especially in the amounts consumed in the United States and other developed countries, poses a significant risk to being diagnosed with cancer. The EPIC-Oxford study is a great example of this. It is one of the largest studies ever conducted, including current and past, to have analyzed the relationship between diet and cancer. Researchers looked at 63,550 men and women and found that the overall incidence of cancer was higher in meat eaters than in those following a plant-based lifestyle.[13] In particular, small but notable higher rates of stomach, lung, breast, ovarian, and prostate cancers were all seen in meat eaters compared to their plant-eating counterparts.

One likely explanation is that individuals who eat a lot of meat typically consume more fat in their diet and end up with a higher BMI on average than plant-based eaters do.[14] This is a big deal and has become increasingly publicized in the media as report after report points to the growing link between obesity and cancer.

The bottom line is that fat equals cancer.[15] The more you have of it, the more types of cancer you're susceptible to. According to the American Institute for Cancer Research there's convincing evidence linking higher levels of body fat to cancers of the esophagus, pancreas, colon and rectum, breasts (postmenopausal), endometrium, and kidneys.[16]

The typical Western diet consists of 20 to 35 percent of its calories from fat and much of this is from animal sources. An individual following a healthy, plant-based lifestyle consumes only 7 to 15 percent of calories from fat. Plant-based sources of fat (such as that found in nuts, seeds, and avocados) are also accompanied by a healthy dose of fiber and a multitude of antioxidants and phytonutrients. All of these additional nutritional components in plant foods are a bonus in fighting cancer and preventing the growth of malignant cells.

Numerous studies have linked the consumption of meat and cancer. I highlight just a few:

- Higher levels of meat, especially red meat (beef, pork, and lamb) and processed meat (hot dogs, chicken nuggets, lunch meats, bacon, cured/salted meats), are associated with higher rates of colorectal, esophageal, lung, pancreatic, endometrial, stomach, and prostate cancer.[17]
- Grilling, frying, or barbecuing meats leads to the formation of potent carcinogenic compounds known as heterocyclic amines (HCAs). HCAs are found in all well-done meats including red meats, chicken, and fish resulting in elevated risks for colon, prostate, and breast cancers.[18] HCAs are also the same toxic chemicals found in tobacco smoke and diesel exhaust.
- Consuming chicken with skin intact has been shown to increase the *progression* of prostate cancer in men by twofold after diagnosis.[19] This may be due in part to two factors. First, chicken is known for forming the highest amounts of HCAs after being cooked, more than any other form of meat. Second, chicken, with the skin, has a much higher fat content than chicken without the skin or even some cuts of red meat.

This evidence presents a startlingly clear message—meat consumption *does not* promote a cancer-free life. If anything it does the opposite. What I've noticed most throughout the years is there are never any headlines in the media or scientific world urging us to consume more meat in order to prevent or reverse cancer. No scientist, no doctor, and no researcher has ever published a study showing that cancer can be beaten by eating more meat. While plenty of studies show a reduced risk of cancer with the consumption of leaner meats, is this really what you want for yourself and your family?

> Winning the war on cancer doesn't mean less cancer. Winning the war on cancer means no cancer.

Winning the war on cancer doesn't mean less cancer. Winning the war on cancer means no cancer. To do this, animal-based proteins are best left at the farm where they came from and not given a place at your dinner table.

Starving Cancer

Animal-based proteins and fats play significant roles in jump starting cancer growth, but they're not the only dietary factors at work in this deadly disease. Two additional factors are critical for the continued growth, progression, and metastasis (spread) of cancer.

The first includes the process of angiogenesis. Angiogenesis is the formation of new blood vessels around the cancerous tumor. The second involves the consumption of added sugars in one's diet, which helps feed and accelerate tumor growth. Gaining an understanding of these concepts will help you understand what to do and what not to do in order to avoid a grueling battle with cancer. Starving cancer begins with eliminating animal-based and processed foods first and is continued by replacing them with antioxidant-rich, plant-based foods.

Preventing Angiogenesis Through Dietary Means

Cancer cells are just like any other living cell. They need fuel (that is, nutrients) to survive and grow. These nutrients are delivered to them via the blood supply just like any other cell in the body receives nutrients. Yet unlike other cells in the body, cancer cells need *a lot* of nutrients in order to overpower and invade adjacent healthy tissue. The only way to accomplish this is to build a large network of blood vessels capable of supplying a massive amount of nutrients to feed an accelerated rate of growth.

This process is known as tumor angiogenesis. Think of it as the equivalent of a baseball player who wants to be the home run king but doesn't have the strength and power to do so. The player enlists the help of some shady individuals who have the ability to get him what he needs— steroids and growth hormones. In the case of cancer cells, the "steroids and growth hormones" are primarily glucose molecules (sugar), and the individuals supplying them are the vast network of blood vessels forming around the tumor.

Whether or not a microscopic cluster of cancer cells stays dormant or grows into a massive malignant tumor is largely determined by their ability to successfully undergo tumor angiogenesis. Under normal conditions the body has a number of checks and balances in place to keep the growth of new blood vessel formation under control.[20] In individuals with cancer, however, these various regulators of angiogenesis are damaged by mutant cancer genes rendering them unable to properly carry out their duties.[21]

This leads to an out-of-control explosion of new blood vessel formation to an immature group of cancer cells ensuring their future development into full-blown virulent tumors. This proliferation also provides the network of blood vessels necessary for the cancer to spread to organs and tissues located throughout the body—a process known as metastasis.

Tumor angiogenesis can be curtailed or even stopped though. Antiangiogenic treatments are currently being developed and tested by pharmaceutical companies to suppress the rate of tumor angiogenesis in cancer patients. Unlike conventional cancer treatments, which target both cancerous and healthy cells, antiangiogenic medications zero in on much more specific targets and thus do not have nearly the amount of severe, debilitating side effects as chemotherapeutic agents. This does not mean they are without side effects though. These agents have been known to cause elevated blood pressure, excess protein in the urine, serious bleeding events, blood clots, impaired wound healing, and other serious adverse events.

Although antiangiogenic therapies offer an additional or alternative treatment course to conventional approaches to fighting cancer, we still have a lot to learn about these agents in the years to come before they become standard of care. More information is available at the Angiogenesis Foundation's website at www.angio.org if you wish to explore the topic further.

What I find remarkable is that antiangiogenic properties are already available to us right now. They're in the foods we eat, and they don't come with all of the side effects that their man-made pharmaceutical counterparts do.

Dr. William Li first brought this to the attention of the medical world when he gave his TED2010 lecture in Long Beach, California. In this speech he emphasized how fruits, vegetables, and other whole foods play an integral role in our fight against cancer. His talk can be nicely summed up by this quote from his speech: "The obvious thing is to think about what we could remove from our diet. But I took a completely opposite approach and began asking: What could we be adding to our diet that could boost the body's defense system? In other words, can we eat to starve cancer?"[22]

It turns out we can eat to starve cancer by suppressing tumor angiogenesis with health-promoting, plant-based whole foods. An article published by Dr. Li in the *Journal of Oncology* explains in detail which foods suppress tumor angiogenesis and which cancers they specifically target.[23] The chart provided on the next page outlines Dr. Li's findings.

Cancer's Drug of Choice—Sugar

Cellular metabolism is at the core of sustaining life. For normal, healthy cells this process occurs every millisecond of every day without a problem.

Antiangiogenic Properties of Various Dietary Sources

Antiangiogenic Agent(s)	Food Item(s)	Targeted Cancers
Polyphenol catechins	Green tea	Colon, prostate, lung, esophageal, oral, cervical
Genistein	Soybeans	Breast, prostate
Resveratrol	Mulberries, peanuts, grapes, grape products, red and rose wines	Breast, prostate, skin, lung
Lycopene	Tomatoes, watermelon, papaya	Breast, prostate, liver, colon
Omega-3 fatty acids	Flax seed, chia seeds, walnuts	Breast, bone, pancreatic, colon, prostate
Glucosinolates, Isothiocyanates, Indole-3-carbinol	Cruciferous vegetables (cabbage, broccoli, kale)	Lung, oral, pharynx, larynx, esophageal, non-Hodgkin's lymphoma, ovarian
Quercetin	Dark leafy greens, onions	Lung, colorectal, prostate, ovarian, laryngeal, esophageal, gastric
Anthocyanins	Berries, grapes	Esophageal, oral
Proanthocyanidins	Cacao, cinnamon, cranberry, apples, grapes, black current, persimmons	Melanoma, liver, lung, colorectal, oral, laryngeal, breast, ovarian, non-Hodgkin's lymphoma
Circumin	Turmeric spice	Skin, stomach, colon, liver, prostate, bladder
Ellagitannins	Pomegranate, walnuts, pecans, strawberries, blackberries, raspberries	Prostate
Menaquinone	Natto (fermented soy)	Lung, prostate, liver
Beta-cryptoxanthin	Orange, red, and yellow fruits and vegetables	Cervical, lung, gall bladder, breast

Cancer cells are different though. The DNA of cancer cells has been permanently mutated or damaged causing individual components within these cells to act out inappropriately. Consequently, a supercharged metabolic process ensues that puts cellular activity into overdrive. This flurry of activity produces far too many new cells and inhibits the death of old cells—defined as apoptosis—resulting in the growth of a malignant tumor.[24]

Since cancer cells have the ability to thrive in an environment with or without oxygen, the key to their being able to sustain a high level of metabolism is found within a continuous supply of nutrients. The nutrient of choice for cancer cells is *sugar*. Cancer cells are addicted to sugar much like a drug addict is addicted to their drug of choice. When sugar is consumed in the diet, especially added sugars and/or refined carbohydrates, it feeds cancer growth.

> Cancer cells are addicted to sugar much like a drug addict is addicted to their drug of choice.

Eating small amounts of sugar found naturally in fruits and vegetables (carrots, apples, oranges, bananas, for example) is normally not a problem. The problem arises when individuals with advanced stages of cancer undergo the extensive process of tumor angiogenesis. As you recall from the previous section, this is the lifeline that cancerous growths are counting on to ensure their survival. Consuming large amounts of added sugars or refined carbohydrates provides a steady influx of glucose for these sugar-craving cancer cells to gorge on allowing them to grow limitlessly in their quest to take over the human body.

The transformation of these large amounts of sugar into usable energy is accomplished through a process known as glycolysis, but there's a hitch with cancer cells. Since cancer cells don't operate in the same manner as healthy cells, they need significantly more glucose to meet their demands.[25] As a result, cancerous tumors uptake much larger quantities of available glucose in the body compared to normal cells. This heightened degree of glucose uptake has actually been used to analyze the extent of disease progression and remission in cancer patients as well as their future prognosis. Tumors demonstrating a larger uptake of glucose, via positron emission tomography imaging (the PET scan), carry a poorer prognosis in terms of survival time than tumors uptaking less glucose into their cells.[26]

The increased utilization of glucose in cancer cells eventually leads to tumorigenesis—formation of new tumors. Three main things take place to make this a reality. These three processes are what help further support cellular proliferation and the eventual metastasis of cancer throughout the rest of the body.[27]

- **Continued glucose uptake.** Cancer cell glycolysis supports a continual feeding frenzy of glucose molecules upon itself. A similar concept would be to envision an individual attending an all-you-can-eat buffet with a malfunctioning hunger switch inside of them. Not only does this hunger switch fail to tell the individual when to stop eating, but it's always turned on so they continue to stuff themselves day after day until they become so morbidly obese they eventually completely debilitate themselves and cause their own demise.

- **Suppression of apoptosis.** Apoptosis is programmed cell death. It's nature's way of shipping out the old and bringing in the new. Cancerous tumors are able to effectively slow down or stop this process ensuring their continued growth, takeover, and destruction of the host they inhabit.

- **Increased production of fatty acids.** During cancer cell glycolysis some glucose is converted into energy, but some is turned into little particles of fat called fatty acids. Normally, these fatty acids are metabolized by the mitochondria (powerhouses of the cell) to extract energy from them. However, in cancer cells these fatty acids are often used to help form cell membranes in new, rapidly dividing cells. This, once again, helps cancer cells rapidly grow and divide, further promoting the progression of the cancer itself.

If you avoid both added sugars and refined carbohydrates in your diet, your body has the ability to stop the out-of-control glucose feast that occurs during the progression of cancer. This is an absolute must for anyone suffering from the disease and is a good habit to get into for anyone wishing to prevent cancer.

In a culture and society that's inundated with so many sugary foods, be it hidden or unhidden forms of sugar, this is easier said than done. But if you wish to give yourself the best possible chance of remaining cancer free, the question that begs asking is are those daily fixes of white bread, white pasta, soda pop, rich desserts, and other highly concentrated sources of sweeteners worth all the pain and suffering endured during the course of battling cancer?

Only you can answer this question for yourself. I hope the answer is no. I hope you can find a healthier, more natural way of getting your sweet kicks the next time the glucose fairy comes calling. Chef AJ's story will really bring this all home to you, as she was a sweetaholic.

Chef AJ's Story

Abbie Jaye, better known as Chef AJ, is the epitome of healthy eating. She also just so happens to be one of the most masterful creators of wholesome, delicious raw/vegan pastries in all of North America, and she pulls it off without using any processed foods. Her culinary delights, along with her incredible story, can be found in her book Unprocessed, which I deem a must-read for any food lover or health enthusiast.

Her climb to the top as a promoter of a sustainable, healthy way of life wasn't always easy though. Chef AJ had to fight an endless stream of battles along the way to get where she is today. One of those battles included overcoming her worst addiction—sugar!

Chef AJ's struggles began in early childhood when she became overweight. Constantly teased and ridiculed, she took these jabs and insults personally and became severely depressed because of them. She eventually became anorexic as her way of coping with the bullying. Anorexia would be her crutch for eleven long years. During those critical developmental adolescent and young adulthood years, anorexia literally brought her to the brink of death as she was hospitalized for a period of several months during the middle of her college career.

Once she overcame this terrible disorder, Chef AJ didn't just start eating again, she started bingeing. Unfortunately, she ate with a vengeance and resorted to the worst possible foods she could find—loads of processed junk foods. Ice cream, pastries, candy, and everything in between filled her daily menu. Over the years Chef AJ would continue to battle her childhood weight problems and eventually became obese again. She gained sixty pounds from her anorexic low and developed a severe case of adult-onset asthma. This required a myriad of prescription drugs to treat.

Chef AJ was technically a vegetarian at this point in her life and would later become a full-fledged vegan. Even at this, though, her diet was abominable at best. Full of calories and devoid of nutrients was the perfect way to describe her diet. Chef AJ's asthma would finally disappear only to be replaced by other more pressing health concerns. Her vegan diet consisted of three basic food groups—fat, sugar, and salt—none of which were doing her any good. She would soon experience multiple miscarriages, suffer from another bout of depression, and eventually develop severe anxiety leading to numerous panic disorders in the coming years.

After the heartbreaking loss of her beloved pet dog, the death of her mother and father, and hearing the devastating news from her doctor that she'd never be able to have kids due to the multiple operations she underwent to address her previous reproductive problems, Chef AJ completely broke down and turned to food once again. Her sugar addiction "went through the roof" at this point as she recalls in her book.[28] Her diet went from bad to worse as she regularly downed 32-ounce Coke Slurpees and 48-ounce Big Gulps for her daily breakfasts and lunches.

Then in 2003 on New Year's Day one of her worst nightmares came true. As she was attempting to have a bowel movement, a sea of blood filled her toilet as she bled profusely, igniting a fear that rocked her to the core. Chef AJ was terrified by the instant thought of colon cancer as this had run in her family. Colon cancer had taken the life of her grandmother.

She consulted her doctor as soon as possible and underwent a sigmoidoscopy only to find out what she had hoped was never true—a diagnosis of bleeding adenomatous polyps in the sigmoid colon. These are the precancerous types of polyps that almost always develop into full-blown colon cancer given enough time, especially when there's a strong family history of it.[29]

Chef AJ had had enough at this point. She was not going to be another statistic. Instead, she decided to make a choice. One that would dramatically change her lifestyle as she chose food over medicine, utensils over scalpels, and a long-term solution over a short-term fallacy.

Chef AJ would enter the Optimum Health Institute's (OHI) program in San Diego. OHI, much like the Hippocrates Health Institute in West Palm Beach, Florida, specializes in healing individuals with a 100 percent organic, raw foods diet. They do it by offering a variety of fruits, vegetables, sprouts, and freshly made vegetable juices to their clients. They also eliminate animal-based and processed foods.

This diet would be an enormous challenge for Chef AJ because processed foods were the staple of her regular diet. She struggled for days as her body detoxed off the vegan junk foods she'd been consuming. As her cravings for these toxic foods disappeared, they were eventually replaced by an appreciation for the life-giving properties of healthy, plant-based whole foods. This was the new lease on life Chef AJ had always been looking for, and it was healing her body with each new day.

Six months after leaving OHI she went back to her doctors for a follow-up sigmoidoscopy. To their disbelief her precancerous polyps had vanished completely! They were replaced by vibrant pink walls of a normal, healthy colon. Chef AJ had beaten cancer before it had even had a chance to start.

To this day she continues to follow this lifestyle and includes a variety of fruits, vegetables, lentils, and whole grains in her daily diet. She's finally back in control of her own life and now finds joy in transforming the lives of others by teaching them about the powerful properties of real food—bright, colorful, unprocessed whole foods.

The Moss Reports

Before concluding this chapter I would be remiss if I didn't mention the incredible work of Ralph Moss, PhD. Dr. Moss is a medical writer who has spent over forty years of his career researching and writing about cancer and cancer-related therapies including both conventional (chemotherapy, radiation, surgery) as well as alternative forms of treatment (nutritional, homeopathic, watchful waiting, and others). He has written or edited twelve books and three film documentaries on cancer research and treatment, including the award-winning PBS documentary *The Cancer War*. He is also the former science writer and assistant director of public affairs at the Memorial Sloan-Kettering Cancer Center in New York, one of the world's premier cancer centers. He has a brilliant mind and is highly respected for his life's work in cancer and cancer-related research.

Dr. Moss has compiled what is known as *The Moss Reports*—a comprehensive review of the twenty-five most common types of cancers and their available treatments (both conventional and alternative) along with the success rates of these treatments. His reports are evidence-based and incorporate what he has learned as he's traveled the globe studying and speaking to the leading experts and physicians in the field of cancer. He has made these reports available for a reasonable fee at CancerDecisions.com to help those facing this disease, along with their doctors, in hopes of giving them a better understanding of *all* available options when treating specific cancer diagnoses.

This service may not seem valuable to you at first but realize that the healthcare practitioner currently treating you is likely to do what anyone would do in their shoes—offer the information and knowledge they've gathered throughout their life experience of treating patients with cancer. This means if your doctor attended medical school, he or she will most likely inform you of your options using chemotherapy, radiation, or surgical methods used to treat cancer. If your doctor attended an alternative or holistic medical school, then you'll likely be informed of your options in using alternative medical therapies to treat cancer. Both doctors are doing their absolute best to treat you, and both may have valuable information when it comes to treating this disease. But both may not be aware of all available treatment options and their current success rates.

This is where Dr. Moss comes in. His work provides a roadmap, so to speak, in helping you and your doctor better understand these options to help you decide which choice(s) gives you the best possible chance of improving cancer remission rates, increasing survival time, and providing the best quality of life during and after treatment. This type of information is invaluable in my opinion and well worth the time and resources needed to investigate it, especially in the wake of a life-and-death disease.

Autoimmune Diseases

"We put drugs of which we know little, into bodies
of which we know less, to cure diseases
of which we know nothing at all."

—VOLTAIRE

L ike any other day, April 11, 1861, began with a serene sense of calmness as the waters off Charleston Harbor barely made a ripple in Fort Sumter, South Carolina. This would be the last day peace and solitude would embrace this city as the United States would soon be at war with itself the very next day. April 12 dawned the only civil war America has ever experienced as soldiers from the North and South violently clashed with one another over the highly contentious antislavery movement brought about by the 1860 presidential election of Abraham Lincoln. This type of self-inflicted pain for a nation of people is out of the ordinary, and it resulted in the deadliest war the United States has ever participated in as casualties exceeded 600,000.

Much like this dark side of American history, it is also out of the ordinary for our body to attack itself, but this is exactly what happens in the case of an autoimmune disease. The human body wages civil war against

Partial List of Autoimmune Disorders	
Celiac Disease	Type 1 Diabetes
Grave's Disease	Scleroderma
Psoriasis	Ulcerative Colitis
Rheumatoid Arthritis	Crohn's Disease
Myasthenia Gravis	Sjögren's Syndrome
Multiple Sclerosis	Addison's Disease
Hashimoto's Thyroiditis	Systemic Lupus Erythematosus

itself as it targets its own cells, tissues, and organs with an immune system raging out of control. While the origins and complexities of more than eighty different autoimmune disorders are not completely understood yet, what is known is that genetic makeup accounts for only 25 to 40 percent of disease risk while environmental influences account for the remainder.[1]

What you eat or don't eat plays a huge role in this process. Adopting a whole foods, plant-based lifestyle can dramatically reduce the pain and suffering experienced by those with one of these diseases. In some cases a change in lifestyle and eating can even reverse the disease if caught early enough. I will cover a few of the more common autoimmune diseases that respond best to nutritional interventions and lifestyle medicine in this chapter.

Multiple Sclerosis

Multiple sclerosis (MS) affects up to 2.5 million people worldwide and an estimated 400,000 people in the United States.[2,3] Women are affected more than men, and the average age of onset is between twenty and forty years old. The disease affects the central nervous system with 85 percent of initial cases being defined as relapsing-remitting. Patients begin by experiencing episodes of acute attacks followed by periods of improvement. Eventually, these individuals will experience a gradual, slow decline in their overall physical health due to disease progression. However, most live an average lifespan despite this fact, totaling thirty-five years or longer after the onset of initial symptoms.

The progression of MS is characterized by an autoimmune inflammatory response, which destroys the myelin sheath surrounding the nerve fibers of the brain and spinal cord.[4] This myelin sheath is responsible for protecting and insulating the body's nerve cells as well as facilitating the transmission of electrochemical messages from one nerve cell to another. When this protective layer of myelin surrounding the nerves is damaged, it diminishes the body's ability to receive and send messages resulting in loss of function and a number of debilitating symptoms. These symptoms include numbness, tingling, vision disturbances, dizziness, muscle weakness, fatigue, nerve pain, and cognitive dysfunction. Moderate disability usually results within ten years of being diagnosed with MS, and patients often eventually use a wheelchair or become bedridden after an average of twenty-eight years of being diagnosed.[5]

Modern medicine has little to offer in treating MS. There are a small number of medications called disease-modifying drugs (DMDs) used as first-line agents to help delay the progression of MS. These include Copaxone, Tysabri, and various Interferon beta products (Avonex, Betaseron, Rebif). These drugs are very expensive (as high as $25,000 per year) and have not been proven to reduce long-term disability outcomes in MS.[6,7]

At best, these drugs are simply a bandage and come with some risky side effects. Some of the side effects include a weakened immune system leading to frequent or severe infections, flu-like symptoms, depression (including suicidal thoughts), bleeding disorders, heart problems such as chest pain and high blood pressure, and thyroid dysfunction. While some patients do get temporary relief with these agents, a much safer and more effective way of treating MS is with plant-based nutrition.

Roy Swank, MD, led the way with this research. He dedicated his entire life to defeating multiple sclerosis and accumulated more than fifty years of research on diet and MS. He found nutrition outshined the modern "miracles" of medications in every single instance when his patients remained compliant with his program.

Dr. Swank used a very low-fat, plant-based diet to reduce the amount, frequency, and severity of attacks in his patients suffering from MS. Dr. Swank's menu for his patients consisted of generous amounts of fruits, vegetables, and whole grains along with small amounts of meat, low-fat dairy products, nuts and seeds, and vegetable oils. The key to his success was limiting both total and saturated fat intake. He allowed no more than 15 grams of saturated fat and 20 to 50 grams of total fat per day. The less fat the better, according to Dr. Swank. If you compare this to the typical fast food meal of American pizza, it doesn't take long for someone to reach their limit using Dr. Swank's guidelines. Two slices of medium, hand-tossed, Pepperoni Lover's® pizza from Pizza Hut contain a total of 26 grams of fat and 12 grams of saturated fat.[8]

In 1990, Dr. Swank published the results from his MS research in the prestigious medical journal *The Lancet*. In this report, he noted that patients following his low-fat diet had a 95 percent chance of surviving and remaining physically active after a thirty-four-year period.[9] These results were unheard of in conventional medicine at the time, and still are today even with all the new blockbuster drugs available.

Here's a case in point: A 2012 study on those receiving one of the most common medications used to treat MS—Interferon beta—found a death reduction rate of only 46.8 percent after a twenty-one-year period of taking the medication.[10] This is less than half the rate of success of Dr. Swank's approach. It also comes at a much larger cost considering both the financial cost (an estimated $25,000 per year) and side-effect profile with this type of medication.

John McDougall, MD, author of *The Starch Solution*, is another expert physician pioneering research in the field of nutrition and MS. He has taken Dr. Swank's diet and kicked it up a notch by excluding all animal-based foods and vegetable oils. Dr. McDougall uses a starch-based diet with large amounts of fruits and vegetables to achieve similar, if not better, results than Dr. Swank in his patients suffering from MS.

He has found that the earlier the patients start on this nutritional plan, the better their prognosis. The absence of animal-based protein, in particular dairy products, seems to have a substantial effect on those suffering with MS. Many studies have shown the risk of MS, much like type 1 diabetes, significantly increases in those who consume large amounts of milk in their childhood

> The absence of animal-based protein, in particular dairy products, seems to have a substantial effect on those suffering with MS.

years.[11] It is thought that the proteins found in dairy mimic the myelin proteins surrounding the nerve cells in MS patients, causing the body to identify these proteins as foreign, and subsequently attacking the nerve cells because of this.

The outstanding work spanning several decades of both Dr. Swank and Dr. McDougall has proven that keeping it simple provides the best alternative to modern medicine when treating MS. Adopting a whole foods, plant-based lifestyle can be a life changer for those with the disease and should be the first line of therapy in approaching multiple sclerosis.

Rheumatoid Arthritis

Rheumatoid arthritis (RA) is an autoimmune disease that causes inflammation of the joints and surrounding tissues, particularly in the hands, wrists, feet, and knees. Morning joint stiffness, fatigue, and pain are some of the first signs of the disease. Over time joints can lose their range of motion and become permanently deformed leading to severe disability. In addition, advanced cases of RA are linked with other serious health problems such as cardiovascular disease, infections, and depression.[12] Due to the debilitating nature of this chronic disease, it is important to seek and implement adequate treatment interventions as early as possible to prevent permanent joint destruction.

Modern medicine's first line of therapy for patients with RA most often involves medications. Disease-modifying antirheumatic drugs (DMARDs), such as methotrexate and leflunomide, are typically the first to be prescribed. These medications work by reducing inflammation and slowing the progression of the disease. However, they provide minimal relief at best and are extremely toxic at worst. Methotrexate is the most common DMARD used in treating RA resulting in remission rates of 44 percent after six months and 32 percent after two years.[13]

Keep in mind RA lasts for decades and four of every five patients who start DMARD therapy will have discontinued this therapy within five years because of the toxic side effects of these drugs.[14]

Methotrexate is littered with side effects, many of which are extremely serious. This shouldn't come as a surprise considering methotrexate is also a chemotherapy agent used to treat various forms of cancer. Its side effects include damage to the lining of the stomach and intestines, headaches, confusion, blurred vision, liver disease, mouth sores, hair loss, blood cell disorders, severe lung damage, and decreased immune function leading to increased infections.[15,16]

Another line of treatment for RA is nonsteroidal anti-inflammatory drugs (NSAIDs such as ibuprofen and naproxen) and corticosteroids (prednisone). These are commonly prescribed to reduce inflammation in patients with RA. Like DMARD therapy these agents only provide temporary relief and come with a host of adverse effects. NSAIDs have the potential to cause fluid retention and upset stomach and increase the risk of developing bleeding ulcers.

Prednisone has both short- and long-term side effects. Short-term side effects include stomach irritation, sleep disturbances, weight gain, and mood changes. Long-term side effects include increased risk of osteoporosis, atherosclerosis, high blood pressure, Cushing's syndrome, cataracts, glaucoma, stomach ulcers, and increased infections due to a weakened immune system.[17]

The drugs I've mentioned up to this point are all older medications typically used to treat RA. A newer line of agents called biological agents is now available for those who have more advanced cases of RA. These agents (Humira, Enbrel, and Remicade, to name a few) are incredibly expensive averaging $17,000 to $18,000 per year and have not currently shown any long-term measure of success in treating RA.[18] Like DMARDs, they only serve to provide short-term relief of symptoms while delaying the progression of the disease.

The number one drawback to these agents is their potential to increase the chance of serious infections. Biologic agents do this by suppressing the body's own immune system rendering it incapable of fighting off harmful viral and bacterial infectious organisms. One group of biologics, known as TNF (tumor necrosis factor) alpha inhibitors, carry a twofold increased risk of serious infections, such as pneumonia and blood-borne bacterial infections.[19,20] This is a stiff price to pay for subpar therapy.

A much safer, and arguably more effective way, to treat RA is through the healing powers of plant-based, whole foods. Dr. Joel Fuhrman has been doing this for years with incredible success in his patients. He has conducted medically supervised, water-only fasts for one to three weeks in patients with RA, followed by a transition to a menu of nutrient-rich, plant-based foods including fruits, vegetables, legumes, and nuts and seeds.[21] His patients were able to discontinue their medications and experience dramatic reductions in joint pain and stiffness resulting in months or even years of relief as long as they continued to follow this lifestyle change. Some of Dr. Fuhrman's patients have also experienced complete remission of RA by adopting this approach, all without the toxic side effects of taking medications.

These same benefits were seen in a review of thirty-one studies looking at a period of fasting followed by a vegetarian diet in patients with RA.[22] Four studies from this group showed a "statistically and clinically signifi-cant beneficial long-term effect" in treatment of RA. One study in partic-ular looked at the effect of how different foods, when added back into the diet, affected patients over a two-year period.[23]

Participants initially followed a health-centered, vegetarian diet for thirteen months. After this period, some patients opted to add meat and other processed foods back into their diet. Fifty-nine percent of patients reported an increase in disease symptoms when meat was added back into the diet, and 45 percent reported an increase in symptoms when sugar and coffee were reintroduced into the diet. These results stress the importance of maintaining a whole foods, plant-based lifestyle for those RA patients wanting to remain symptom free and in good health.

Systemic Lupus Erythematosus

Another autoimmune disease that can mimic the severe joint pain seen in rheumatoid arthritis is systemic lupus erythematosus (SLE). This disorder usually affects women of childbearing age with the peak age of onset being between the late teens and mid-forties.[24] Lupus can also affect men, but to a much lesser extent.

Early signs of the disease include general fatigue, swollen lymph nodes, headaches, mouth sores, sensitivity to sunlight, skin rashes, chest pains, fever, hair loss, and joint pain/swelling of the fingers, hands, wrists, and knees. It is truly a debilitating illness.

It's important that this disease be diagnosed as early as possible due to the severe, sometimes permanent damage that can take place in major organ systems throughout the body. Advanced stages of lupus can result in life-threatening blood clots, miscarriages, various blood cell disorders, kidney failure, fluid buildup around the heart and lungs, seizures, and even psychiatric disorders resulting in frequent episodes of delusions and hallucinations.

One major concern affecting many lupus sufferers is the development of severe atherosclerosis during the course of the disease. Accelerated atherosclerosis is 2.5 times more prevalent in patients with lupus compared to those without the disease.[25] This arterial plaque buildup can have dire consequences for a person's cardiovascular system and can even lead to premature death from a heart attack or stroke.

The cause of lupus is not completely known at this time. However, it is known both genetics and environmental triggers determine disease risk.[26] Women of African, Native American, and Asian descent have a higher prevalence of the disease compared to those of European descent. Other factors such as smoking, exposure to environmental toxins, and childhood infections can play a role. Diet is also a major determining factor in whether or not individuals will experience signs and symptoms of SLE.

With all this being said, the one thing everyone with lupus shares in common, much like all autoimmune diseases, is the fact that the body develops antibodies against its own cells and tissues.[27] This essentially "marks" the cell or tissue as a foreign substance and provokes the body to attack itself. For people with lupus this marking can be any cell or any tissue in the body and is the reason why damage is so widespread.

Current treatments for SLE rely heavily on drugs to relieve symptoms or delay the progression of the disease. These prescribed drugs *do not* target the cause of the disease. First-line agents include hydroxychloroquine, a drug used to treat malaria, as well as NSAIDs (such as ibuprofen or naproxen) and corticosteroids (prednisone and methylprednisolone).[28] All of these first-line agents are ordinarily used for mild forms of the disease or for acute flare-ups.

Hydroxychloroquine is typically the first medication prescribed for lupus. Even though hydroxychloroquine is considered one of the safer choices in this line up of drugs, it has potential adverse effects. These commonly include diarrhea, dizziness, stomach cramps, nausea, loss of appetite, and headaches. Although rare, a serious disease of the eye called retinopathy, along with other vision problems, can occur with hydroxychloroquine making it important for users to undergo routine eye exams to monitor for such effects.[29]

Other medications used to treat lupus include immunosuppressive agents such as cyclophosphamide, azathioprine, and Cellcept. These agents can help maintain remission in lupus and are often used in combination with steroids. However, since these medications suppress the immune system, individuals are at a higher risk of getting bacterial and viral infections. This causes concern for doctors and patients alike because both steroids and immunosuppressive agents enhance the risk of serious infections. Of the immunosuppressive medications, cyclophosphamide has the greatest potential to cause side effects, which include infertility issues, blood in the urine, and an increased risk of cancer. Methotrexate is another agent in this group used to treat resistant cases of joint pain and skin disease in lupus.

Ultimately, advanced cases of lupus failing to respond to traditional therapy are typically treated with biological agents (Rituximab, Interferon-alpha). While some reduction in symptoms have been noted in the short term using these agents, the long-term effects are unknown due to a lack of sufficient studies.[30] As mentioned in the previous section on RA, the biggest downfall in using these drugs is the increased risk of serious infections such as pneumonia, tuberculosis, and other major infections.

The good news in all of this is that current therapies have increased five-year survival rates in patients with SLE to more than 90 percent.[31] The bad news is there are no major improvements in complications due to the disease or survival rates beyond the ten-year mark. The better news is there's a far more effective and safer way to treat lupus. This involves adopting a whole foods, plant-based lifestyle. As he did for his patients who suffer from RA, Dr. Fuhrman has successfully treated and even reversed lupus in patients using a vegetable-based diet that omits animal-based and processed foods.[32] Again, there are no side effects to this approach, and it's as simple as changing what one eats.

A review of multiple scientific studies shows why a plant-based diet is so beneficial and why the Standard American Diet can contribute to this dreadful disease. Beneficial and aggravating factors are listed from this review to help you understand why it is so important to adopt a plant-based lifestyle to reduce or eliminate the debilitating effects of lupus:[33]

Aggravating Factors
- Excessive amounts of protein
- Excessive amounts of calories
- Saturated fats
- High amounts of omega-6 fatty acids

Beneficial Factors
- Vitamin E, vitamin A (beta-carotene), and selenium
- Omega-3 fatty acids
- Flaxseed

All the aggravating factors listed are exactly what make up the rich Western diet, while all of the beneficial factors are what is found in whole, plant-based foods. The take home message is that a menu of nutrient-rich, plant-based whole foods works to treat lupus. For this reason, it should be incorporated into the treatment plans for all lupus patients as first-line therapy. This is the choice Vickie made when treating her case of lupus.

My Story (written by Vickie Hajash)

On October 31, 2005, my father passed away from complications related to an autoimmune disease. Six years later, in September 2011, after many visits to various doctors and numerous lab tests, I was diagnosed with the same disease—systemic lupus with a positive double marker of rheumatoid arthritis. My ANA was 1:40 and very specific for lupus. Likewise, I was experiencing the symptoms related to autoimmune diseases including stiff and painful joints, extreme fatigue, and frequent urinary tract infections.

Since there is no known medical cure for lupus, I was expected to begin a regimen of prescription medications including a very strong steroid called prednisone and hydroxychloroquine sulfate. Stronger medications would be added accordingly as the disease progressed, and other organs such as the kidneys, heart and lungs were very likely to be attacked.

In short, my life changed in an instant and I was devastated. The most difficult thing was telling my husband and son the grim reality— my diagnosis of systemic lupus. It would undoubtedly change their lives too.

I have never been one to take prescription drugs unless I absolutely had to. I have always researched the medications prescribed by my physicians and this time was no different. However, when I read of all the side effects associated with my lupus medications, I was stunned. Knowing that these medications would not cure the disease but simply manage my symptoms, I was not convinced that they were worth taking!

I spoke to one of my doctors regarding my reservations. She got very firm with me and told me in no uncertain terms that I needed to trust her and do what I was told if I wanted to get through this. Immediately, I scheduled a second opinion. Likewise, my second doctor told me that she had no qualms with the prescribed medications and felt that they were safe. In fact, she went on to say she would even feel comfortable enough to prescribe them to her own mother. Obviously, I was on my own in finding healthier alternatives.

I wondered if it were really possible to manage such a severe disease naturally. Near my home is a raw food smoothie business called RAWk Star. I decided to stop in to see what type of food they offered and perhaps speak with someone who could answer my questions regarding foods and the immune system. Little did I know that this information would forever transform my health.

I met the owners (Karen and Adam) who spent many hours discussing raw, organic, vegan diets. Furthermore, they introduced me to Dustin Rudolph [the author of this book] who graciously spent time teaching me the importance of cutting out caffeine, sugars, whites (processed flours, sugars, dairy products and salt), meat and processed foods. They explained that in order to stop a disease in its track, I would have to make a commitment to this new diet as a lifestyle change and adhere to it with fidelity.

They asked what my motivation would be to stay on it when temptation came along? Without hesitation I said, "To grow old with my husband, watch my son graduate from college, dance at his wedding and hold my grandchildren!"

I implemented everything they shared with me. I used a strategy of 90 percent raw and 10 percent lightly cooked vegan recipes. March 2012, I visited the RA specialist to get the results of yet another set of lab tests. Her final comments were as follows: prior positive ANA, now negative and with a negative serologic workup. NO EVIDENCE of lupus. Clinically she [me] is feeling very well with diet and exercise.

To date I am feeling healthy. My energy level has returned, which is wonderful because my husband and I will attend my son's graduation, dance at his wedding and have energy to keep up with future grandchildren.

Inflammatory Bowel Disease

The two major types of inflammatory bowel disease (IBD) include ulcerative colitis (UC) and Crohn's disease (CD). Both involve the body attacking its own digestive tract causing the intestines to become severely inflamed and painful. UC affects only the colon (large intestine); whereas Crohn's disease affects any part of the digestive tract from mouth to anus but typically targets the small and large intestines.

IBD is treated like the previously mentioned autoimmune diseases, relying on a barrage of anti-inflammatory medications, corticosteroids, and biological agents. Various antibiotics are also used to treat infections resulting from complications of the disease. In 30 to 40 percent of patients with UC and 70 to 80 percent of patients with CD surgery will eventually be required due to the failure of the medications to control the disease.[34] These are incredibly dismal results by any standards.

In patients requiring surgery, all or part of the affected bowel is permanently removed. This sometimes results in a surgically placed ostomy pouch in patients. An ostomy pouch is a small bag attached to an opening in the abdomen for the purpose of removing bodily wastes. In essence, it's how these patients excrete bowels since they no longer have a colon.

UC and CD can be managed effectively and even reversed in the early stages of the disease before surgical removal of the bowel is needed. This is done by adopting a whole foods, plant-based lifestyle. An imbalance of "protective" and "harmful" bacteria in the gut is a major cause of both UC and CD.[35] Avoiding the rich Western diet and eating a high-fiber diet consisting of whole, plant-based foods restores this imbalance and can lead to remission in patients with IBD.

A 2010 study provided proof of CD remission even in those eating a semi-vegetarian diet (including small amounts of eggs, milk, and fish).[36] One hundred percent of study participants following a semi-vegetarian diet achieved complete remission of Crohn's disease after one year, and 92 percent remained in remission after two years. These results are incredible, to say the least, and unheard of in conventional medicine. No medication has ever shown such success rates in Crohn's. Furthermore, this study went on to note that animal protein, animal fats, sugar, fast foods, chocolate, and cola drinks along with the decreased intake of fruits and vegetables are all highly correlated with the development of IBD.

Psoriasis

Psoriasis is an autoimmune disease in which the body attacks its own skin cells. It produces red, inflamed, thickened plaques with silvery scales on the surface of the skin, which may occur all over the body.[37] Recurring flare-ups of itchy, painful skin lesions are common in most patients, and up to 11 percent will develop psoriatic arthritis as the disease progresses into the joints.[38] Psoriatic arthritis is the type of arthritis Phil Mickelson, the professional golfer, suffers from.

Conventional medicine once again resorts to drug therapy to control the symptoms of psoriasis without giving much thought to addressing the cause. Topical corticosteroid creams and ointments are used as first-line agents to help alleviate symptoms and heal localized lesions. Steroid creams tend to cause noticeable thinning of the skin, which is one of their most common side effects. Other side effects include stretch marks, skin infections, and glaucoma. These tend to happen with more potent formulations and after prolonged use of topical steroids.

Because discontinuation of topical steroids usually leads to rapid flare-ups, other topical agents are often used in combination to control psoriasis, including Dovonex, Tazorac, Psoriatec, and coal tar. These agents produce only moderate relief and can cause a number of side effects such as staining of the skin (coal tar, Psoriatec), skin irritation (Tazorac, Psoriatec, Dovenox), and even birth defects (Tazorac) if used during pregnancy.

When topical agents aren't enough to control symptoms or if psoriatic arthritis develops in advanced cases of psoriasis, many clinicians will resort to local corticosteroid injections, immunosuppressive drugs, and biological agents. These medications, as you may recall, carry their own set of potential problems including decreased immune function leading to an increased risk of developing serious infections.

Natural and alternative therapies should be considered first and foremost in patients with psoriasis due to their effectiveness and safety. Light therapy with UVB rays or modest daily sun exposure can produce relief with little to no increase in skin cancer risk.[39] You can even purchase (with a doctor's prescription) UVB equipment that can be used at home for ongoing therapy, but it's important to always follow a doctor's instructions when doing so. UVA light therapy is effective in treating psoriasis, but should be used with strong caution as it increases the risk of skin cancer. Stress is also a major exacerbating factor in up to 78 percent of psoriasis sufferers.[40] Stress-relieving activities such as yoga and meditation can be of great help and are side-effect free.

The most underappreciated weapon in combating psoriasis, however, is a healthy diet. Dr. McDougall and Dr. Fuhrman have both had tremendous success in eliminating psoriasis in their patients by helping them adopt a whole foods, plant-based lifestyle. Studies have shown that low-calorie, high-nutrient vegetarian diets exhibit marked improvements in patients with psoriasis.[41] Fasting periods and the adoption of a gluten-free diet may also provide additional benefits to psoriasis sufferers. There are no side effects to taking this approach. Patients who remain committed to living a lifestyle of consuming nutrient-rich, plant-based foods and avoiding animal products (including dairy) and processed foods can remain disease free and avoid medications for most, if not all, of their entire life.

Wrapping It Up

With few exceptions, autoimmune diseases are typically treated inappropriately with a toxic combination of anti-inflammatory drugs, corticosteroids, immunosuppressants, biological agents, and surgical procedures. The resulting short- and long-term adverse effects of these approaches can add a hefty price for the mediocre results they produce.

Although medications and surgeries do deserve some credit for producing symptomatic relief and extending lifespans in certain instances, their overall impact tends to favor the medical and pharmaceutical industries in most cases. Patients remain sick ensuring lifelong customers and a steady stream of profits for both industries.

Early intervention and implementation of a whole foods, plant-based lifestyle produces far better results, without any additional risks to patients already undergoing pain and suffering from life-altering illnesses. Every patient deserves to know about this simple, effective approach when facing a debilitating chronic disease. It's for this reason I feel a sense of deep responsibility as a healthcare professional to share this information with you should you find yourself battling an autoimmune disease. As I've mentioned before, often the simplest approach is the best approach.

The Rest of the Story: Healthy Skin, Eyes, Kidneys, and Brain

"He who cures a disease may be the skillfullest, but
he that prevents it is the safest physician."

—THOMAS FULLER

One of my fondest memories as a kid was awakening at the crack of dawn on a brisk summer morning, packing up my lunch, grabbing the soiled water jug container on the way out the door, and jumping into my father's 4x4 pickup truck. It would be another tagalong day as Pops and I set out on a trail of dirt-filled roads leading to the oil field patches located in the forgotten backlands of the beautiful Montana countryside. I'd spend the entire day doing what every twelve-year-old boy would want to do—run aimlessly through the prairie chasing cottontail rabbits, hunt incessantly for rattlesnake tails, and pick off a string of pop cans with my shiny black BB gun.

Those hot summer days were the perfect way to spend a summer vacation. They were never complete though until my dad and I engaged in the ritual of sitting in the cab of his pickup truck, afternoon snacks in hand, waiting to listen to the iconic voice of Paul Harvey on the radio. Soon it would be time for *The Rest of the Story.*

Paul Harvey will always and forever be known as one of the greatest radio personalities ever to take to the microphone. He could suck you into a story like no other. Paul masterfully presented little-known or forgotten facts about popular subjects. He would always give it a little twist at the end too. Without fail, my father and I would experience that "aha" moment after each one of his shows. We'd then smile at each other as if a stroke of genius had just been injected directly into our ever-growing intellectual library.

While I am no match for the intriguing bits of wisdom Paul Harvey enthralled us with, I do hope to unveil some little-known facts behind a few lesser-known diseases typically forgotten about in everyday conversation. These subjects are bound to affect us at some point in life, be it directly or indirectly via a loved one. You've already learned about the well-publicized issues of heart disease, obesity, cancer, and diabetes in previous chapters of this book. We've explored autoimmune diseases and their unsatisfactory treatments. Now you're about to learn about more common medical conditions (yet they're given less attention by the drug companies) such as cataracts, wrinkles, memory loss, and kidney disease.

Protecting Our Protector—The Human Skin

If you're ever on *Jeopardy!* here's a little-known and underappreciated fact: The largest single organ in the human body is the skin. It accounts for 15 percent of a person's total body weight.[1] The skin has many roles, one of which is protecting us from all sorts of dangers including ultraviolet radiation from the sun, bacteria, viruses, and environmental toxins.[2] It also acts as the primary regulator of body temperature and helps each of us recognize the world around us by serving as our main sensory organ. That's a lot of work for one organ. It requires a lot of support to accomplish these tasks.

One major way this support is provided to our skin is through the food choices we make. What we put on our plates each day plays a big role not only in providing a healthy glow and appearance to our skin, but also in helping carry out its various duties. Even though it may seem quite vain, the world around us envies beautiful looks. Beautiful looks start with beautiful skin. So what could food possibly have to do with beautiful skin?

I didn't think much about this until I noticed my first wrinkle forming after staring aimlessly into the mirror one morning. I'm sure each of you has probably done the same in your late twenties or early thirties. Unfortunately, wrinkles form as we age whether we like it or not. It's kind of like a vehicle with high miles on it; eventually the parts wear out and the replacement pieces never seem to be as good as the original.

Two of the main "parts" that provide the supporting structure of our skin are found in the middle layer of the skin.[3] They are known as collagen and elastin. Collagen acts as a building block for the skin, much like bricks and mortar act like building blocks for a new home. Elastin allows the skin to resume its original shape after being stretched or contracted. You can envision this by picturing a rubber band returning to its original shape after being stretched out.

Wrinkles form when collagen and elastin are damaged by oxidative stress. Oxidative stress is caused by the formation of free radicals. Two of the biggest culprits in free radical formation are smoking and exposure to ultraviolet (UV) radiation.[4,5] By not smoking and avoiding excess sun exposure,

> By not smoking and avoiding excess sun exposure, you can help your body preserve its healthy, wrinkle-free skin for years to come.

you can help your body preserve its healthy, wrinkle-free skin for years to come.

Back to food though. Food also plays a role in reducing wrinkles because of its ability to either increase or decrease the formation of free radicals. A study published in the 2010 *British Journal of Nutrition* looked at this phenomenon.[6] After accounting for differences in age, smoking status, BMI, and lifetime sun exposure, researchers found a significantly lower wrinkling score in those who ate higher amounts of antioxidant-rich, plant-based foods, particularly green and yellow vegetables. On the flip side, those who ate a diet high in saturated fat had higher wrinkling scores. Saturated fat is found in higher quantities in processed foods, meat, and dairy products including cheese and butter.

Other studies have found that specific groups of antioxidants provide protection against wrinkles. Anthocyanins—plant-based nutrients found in blueberries and other purple fruits—are one of these groups. They've been shown to reduce the breakdown of collagen due to UVB sunlight exposure.[7] Another class of antioxidants known as phenolic compounds—found in large amounts in pomegranate fruit—have also been shown to prevent the breakdown of collagen fibers.[8] These phenolic compounds promote the formation of new collagen fibers as well. Being a fruit lover really can pay off for those of us seeking to keep our youthful appearance for years to come.

The prevention of wrinkles does wonders for vanity's sake, but a much more important benefit to consuming antioxidant-rich, plant-based foods is their ability to prevent skin cancer. They do this by preventing free radical damage to the skin.

Skin cancer is the most common form of any type of cancer in the U.S. An estimated 3.5 million people were diagnosed with nonmelanoma skin cancer (NMSC) in 2006 alone.[9] Although rarely lethal, NMSC does have the potential to be deadly. The five-year survival rate is 90.7 percent, according to the National Cancer Institute, which is a better survival rate than most cancers.[10] Even though these odds are good, I'm sure many would agree it would be better not to get skin cancer in the first place.

The easiest way to do this is to avoid excessive exposure to the sun, refrain from using tanning beds, and use sunscreens to prevent UV sunlight from damaging your skin. You can also use food to fight skin cancer. Multiple studies have shown that dietary antioxidant vitamins, minerals, and phytochemicals such as carotenoids, tocopherols, and flavonoids have demonstrated a protective effect against sun-exposed skin damage.[11,12]

When researchers studied dietary patterns and the incidence of a particular type of NMSC known as squamous cell carcinoma (SCC), a 54 percent decrease in tumor risk was seen in individuals with a higher fruit and vegetable intake.[13] Dark leafy greens were shown to have the highest protective effect in these individuals. Conversely, individuals consuming the most meat and fat in their diet showed an increased risk of SCC tumors developing.

If you happen to be diagnosed with NMSC, then chances are the best available choices to rid yourself of the disease come in the form of conventional methods. Failure to treat and remove the cancerous tumor greatly increases the risk of it growing and metastasizing, which could lead to death. The most common treatment used for most NMSC is to surgically remove the tumor. This approach is highly successful with five-year cure rates up to 99 percent, but the down side is that it causes physical deformities and/or scarring in most cases.[14]

Other treatments such as radiation, liquid nitrogen therapy (freezing), and procedures using a scraping and cauterization method can be used to remove cancerous tumors. These methods have success rates of over 90 percent, but they also have the potential to cause physical deformities and scarring much like surgery.

Two topical medications are available for patients with small tumors in low-risk locations. They are Aldara (Imiquimod) and 5-FU (fluorouracil) cream. These creams have to be used for at least three to twelve weeks to be effective. Their true effectiveness is difficult to determine because there is no long-term data. Success rates vary from 25 to 100 percent depending on the type and stage of NMSC tumor present.[15]

Nearly all patients who use these products will experience at least one adverse effect. Approximately 15 to 16 percent will experience scarring. For patients using Aldara, permanent skin discoloration affects up to 67 percent of them. Both agents are also prohibitively costly, especially considering their shaky track record. A six-week course of Aldara costs over $800. An eight-week course of 5-FU costs roughly $500. Total cost for surgical excision usually runs around $400 to $500 total.

No matter which way you look at it, preventing skin cancer through the use of lifestyle medicine (limiting sun exposure, not smoking, eating healthy, and so on) is far more effective and less costly, both financially and physically, than dealing with numerous trips to the doctor and potential disfigurement after getting it. I would hope that blueberries and spinach sound more enticing than slicing and dicing. We don't always put 2 and 2 together in this regard when it comes to the health of our skin, but perhaps it's time we start thinking differently.

The Gift to See

My great grandmother was totally blind in both eyes for her entire adult life. I never had the honor of meeting her, but I remember hearing stories from my grandmother about being raised by my great grandmother. She was a fantastic lady and always tended to her children's needs just like any other loving parent. It's too bad she never got to "see" them grow up like every other parent does with their children.

Being able to see is often taken for granted by most of us. We usually go about our daily lives never giving it a second thought. If something goes wrong, then there's a lot that can be done to correct these problems. I've worn glasses or contacts almost my entire life to correct my astigmatism. However, not all vision problems like astigmatism are out of our control. There are still a staggering number of people who cope with vision problems that are largely preventable—namely, cataracts and macular degeneration.

Age-related cataracts are one of the leading causes of blindness world-wide. They're responsible for 48 percent of blindness globally.[16] Cataracts are described as a clouding over of the lens of the eye. If left untreated, they lead to vision loss or blindness. Although surgery is available to remove cataracts, prevention remains our best weapon. If you've never smoked, you already have a 50 percent lower chance of developing cataracts. If you quit smoking for good, your risk is only 16 percent higher than a person who's never smoked at all. If you're a woman, hormone replacement therapy can increase your risk of cataracts by 25 percent.

What you eat also has a major impact on reducing your risk of cataracts. In 2011, the *American Journal of Clinical Nutrition* reported on the reduction in risk of cataracts within various diet groups.[17] Researchers compared individuals who ate greater than or equal to 3.5 ounces of meat per day to those who ate little or no meat. That much meat is about the size of a deck of cards. Study results showed that those who ate only fish had a 21 percent reduction in cataracts compared to meat eaters. Vegetarians had a 30 percent reduction, and vegans had a 40 percent reduction. This research showed that a clear, progressive decrease in cataracts was seen when less animal foods were consumed.

Age-related macular degeneration is another common and rapidly increasing cause of blindness in the developed world. This, too, is largely due to poor diet and lifestyle behaviors.[18] Macular degeneration results in a loss of a person's central vision making it hard to recognize anything directly in front of them. The disorder is more likely to happen as we age but can be prevented by consuming less fat from animal-based and processed foods and eating more nutrients from whole, plant-based foods.[19] Individuals who do this show a positive association with reduced rates of age-related macular degeneration.

Saving Your Kidneys

In June 2012, I read a story in *The New York Times* about a father giving his daughter a second chance at life by donating one of his kidneys.[20] I couldn't help but think of what an incredible gift this was to receive!

Erika Royer, thirty-one years old, was able to go back to work after receiving a kidney transplant from her father. An advanced stage of lupus had robbed her of both her kidneys. Before her dad's generous donation, Erika was hooked up to a dialysis machine three to four times per week for several hours at a time. This greatly reduced her quality of life. The dialysis machine was doing what her kidneys couldn't do anymore—remove the buildup of "garbage" (excess fluid, toxins, and waste products) from her body.

Dialysis is what many patients with end stage renal disease (ESRD) have to go through in order to stay alive. Without dialysis, death is imminent. With dialysis, patients are afforded the continuation of life but often feel miserable on a regular basis as they battle a constant state of fatigue and sickness. Living without your kidneys changes everything in life. Going to the bathroom becomes a luxury of the past and is replaced by constant visits to doctors, hospitals, and dialysis centers. It's a very difficult way of life.

Erika's father, Radburn Royer, couldn't have been happier for his daughter as she was now free, like any other human being, to go and do as she pleased. She could once again use the bathroom. Everything turned out fine from a medical standpoint for both Erika and her father. However, Royer would soon experience the unintended consequences of his precious gift. When seeking medical insurance, he was denied coverage from a private health insurer because of a "preexisting" condition for only having one kidney. He was also denied coverage of a life insurance policy due to this same reason. At fifty-three years old, Royer had literally given up a kidney only to lose his long-term security and financial stability if something were to happen to him.

Hearing stories like this breaks my heart. I can't help but think of how life could've been much different for both Royer and his daughter Erika had they known there was a different way. If somebody would've just shared with them the benefits of a whole foods, plant-based lifestyle in reversing lupus and preventing kidney disease, then maybe this wouldn't have had to happen.

- Maybe Erika could have spent her time pursuing a career and a family instead of attending dialysis sessions three times a week.
- Maybe our healthcare system might have saved the $68,585 in average annual costs that it takes to provide medical care to someone on dialysis each year.[21]
- Maybe a father could have been planning a family vacation instead of trying to figure out how to obtain healthcare insurance after being penalized for doing the right thing.

In any event, I'm here to tell you that kidney disease *is* largely preventable. You don't have to go through what Erika and her family went through. By adopting a whole foods, plant-based lifestyle, you'll be ensuring yourself a lifetime of regular bathroom privileges. This may not sound all that glamorous now but have these privileges taken away and you might think differently.

Diabetes and hypertension (high blood pressure) are the two major causes of kidney disease worldwide.[22] They take away more people's freedom due to kidney failure than any other diseases on the planet. With few exceptions, these medical conditions are both foodborne illnesses. They are due to a diet of animal-based and processed foods. By adopting a whole foods, plant-based lifestyle, the majority of people with kidney disease could avoid these problems entirely. To understand why, it's important to understand how diet affects the kidneys.

The kidneys' main function is to remove excess fluid and waste products from the body. The main excess waste product needing removed for most people is protein. In the United States the average adult consumes anywhere from 66 to 91 grams of protein per day, more than double the amount needed to meet the body's requirements.[23] This excess protein causes the kidneys to work harder to get rid of it.

Over time this leads to progressive damage of the nephrons (small functional components) within the kidneys.[24] It is estimated that as we age we lose approximately 1 percent of our kidney function each year.[25] Living in a society that adores a protein-rich diet of meat, dairy, eggs, protein shakes, protein bars, and other high-protein foods only compounds the stress put on the kidneys.

Although high-protein diets are a major problem when it comes to developing kidney disease, the type of protein consumed is also important. Plant-based, vegetable proteins have been shown to have less of a detrimental effect on the kidneys compared to animal-based proteins.[26] For those who already have kidney disease, removing animal products and consuming a vegan diet has actually been shown to be beneficial in preventing further damage to the kidneys.[27] However, it is still important to realize that any diet high in protein will continue to stress the kidneys. For this reason, it is important to work with a knowledgeable physician or dietitian if you're suffering from kidney disease in order to ensure appropriate protein levels in your diet.

> **High-protein diets are a major problem when it comes to developing kidney disease.**

Potassium and phosphorus levels can also be dangerously high in those with kidney disease, which can cause severe damage to the heart and may even be fatal. This is another reason it's important to work with a qualified healthcare provider regarding diet and kidney disease.

Kidney stones are another condition linked to the Western diet. The two most common forms of kidney stones are calcium stones (consisting of either calcium phosphate or calcium oxalate) and uric acid stones. Diets high in animal protein and sodium greatly increase the risk of both calcium and uric acid stone formation.[28,29] Animal proteins and salt increase calcium and uric acid concentrations in the urine. Excess urinary calcium and uric acid are two of the major components of kidney stones. Oxalates, another dietary component, are also associated with stone formation. Oxalates are found in plant foods such as rhubarb, spinach, beets, wheat bran, strawberries, nuts, seeds, soy products, chocolate, and tea. So does this mean you need to avoid these healthy foods too?

In order to prevent kidney stones the most important thing is to limit or avoid animal proteins along with excessive sodium. If you continue to have problems with stone formation, then limiting foods with oxalates may help prevent future recurrences of stone formation. You should not avoid plant-based foods with oxalates if you do not have recurrent problems with kidney stones or are otherwise healthy.

Overall, as the intake of fruits, vegetables, and other plant-based foods go up, the incidence of kidney stone formation goes down.[29] Why? Because fruits and vegetables have been shown to increase urinary citrate levels—a process that inhibits the formation of calcium stones in the kidneys.

Bottom line is if you want healthy kidneys then adopt a whole foods, plant-based lifestyle and limit or avoid animal-based and processed foods. This will reduce excess protein and sodium in your diet. It will also replace harmful animal-based proteins with healthier plant-based proteins.

Avoiding Dementia

Both of my grandmothers currently suffer from dementia. One has a diagnosis of Alzheimer's disease (AD) while the other is experiencing memory loss and cognitive impairment. For many families this is an all too common occurrence among their elders. Chances are you can probably relate to this with your own family. Even though dementia is a nonreversible degenerative disease, it is preventable by following a whole foods, plant-based lifestyle focused on nutritional excellence. The earlier you start eating this way, the better the chances of preventing dementia.

Dementia begins with short-term forgetfulness and progresses to stages of confusion, disorientation, impaired judgment, and difficulty communicating. Eventually, patients will no longer be able to carry out activities of daily living (bathing, dressing, eating, using the bathroom). At the final stage, they can even lose the ability to recognize loved ones. Ultimately, dementia is fatal.

Alzheimer's disease, the most common form of dementia, is the sixth leading cause of death in America according to 2011 data from the CDC.[30] The average survival time after onset of dementia is only 4.5 years but can be up to 10.7 years for some individuals.[31] These last years of life are usually of very poor quality. The "long goodbye" often takes a heartbreakingly huge toll, both physically and emotionally, on patients and their loved ones.

There are currently only five FDA-approved medications (Aricept, Cognex, Exelon, Razadyne, and Namenda) for treating Alzheimer's disease. None of them cures or stops the progression of the disease. They only manage to improve symptoms for a minority of people who take them. Only 10 to 20 percent of users will see an improvement in cognition, activities of daily living, and behavioral symptoms during the first six to twelve months while using these medications.[32] After this initial period of time, there is no benefit to taking these drugs.

Shockingly, an even larger proportion of patients (20 to 40 percent) actually get worse and continue to deteriorate while taking these medications. The average cost of just one of these drugs is $1,800 per year.[33]

The best protection against dementia lies with prevention. It's imperative to avoid contributing lifestyle factors such as smoking, excessive alcohol consumption, B vitamin deficiencies, high cholesterol, high blood pressure, and poor diet. The rich Western diet is by far the biggest factor of all of these.

People with higher intakes of saturated and trans fats in their diet experience two to three times the risk of Alzheimer's disease and have faster rates of cognitive decline than their healthier-eating counterparts.[34] Saturated and trans fats are found mostly in meat, dairy, and processed foods (deep fried fast foods, potato chips, pastries). These same foods also significantly raise cholesterol levels. Studies have shown that elevated levels of blood cholesterol during midlife increase the risk of developing AD by as much as threefold.[35,36]

Alzheimer's disease is characterized by the death of brain cells. The death of brain cells is linked primarily to the presence of two substances deposited throughout the diseased brain—neurofibrillary tangles (NFTs) and senile plaques.[37] Senile plaques are made up of a protein called beta-amyloid. It has been shown that dietary fat and cholesterol imbalances increase the formation of both NFTs and senile plaque deposits within the brain.[38] Diets with a greater proportion of fruits and vegetables, on the other hand, provide a protective effect against dementia.[39]

Certain foods in particular have been shown to be beneficial in reducing the incidence of Alzheimer's disease. Antioxidants called polyphenols found in apples, purple grapes, grapefruit, blueberries, and cranberries protect the brain and reduce the risk of AD.[40] Spices such as turmeric and cinnamon also have a preventive effect on AD.

Omega-3's are also of great importance in avoiding AD. Omega-3 fatty acids, specifically docosahexaenoic acid (DHA), has been shown in animal studies to promote the growth of new connections between nerve cells in the brain.[41] This allows for increased capability of nerve cells to communicate with one another thereby improving their overall functioning. A high-DHA diet in animal studies has been shown to decrease the production of beta-amyloid by as much as 70 percent, thus reducing the formation of senile plaques.[42] The best sources for obtaining healthy omega-3's, including DHA, are ground flaxseeds, chia seeds, walnuts, and dark leafy greens. Don't go overboard with the nuts and seeds though. It only takes a mere tablespoon per day to get all the omega-3's your body needs for that day.

I find this information extremely exciting! What once was thought to be a chronic disease of natural aging is now something we can prevent. Dementia and, specifically, AD are largely a product of the same food choices that heart disease and diabetes are. Gravitating away from a rich Western diet and adopting a whole foods, plant-based lifestyle will undoubtedly keep both your heart and your brain functioning at a high level for a long period of time. It's the easiest, simplest side-effect and cost-free form of "medicine" anyone could use in an effort to preserve brain health.

A Look Behind the Scenes of Medicine, Food, and Politics

"Unless we put medical freedom in the Constitution, the time will come when medicine will organize itself into an undercover dictatorship to restrict the art of healing to one class [of people] and deny equal privileges to others."
—DR. BENJAMIN RUSH

Few medical discoveries truly have a significant impact on society as a whole. When these occur, we often are not aware of their significance immediately. It may take years before any positive effect is seen in the public arena from these discoveries. The practice of lifestyle medicine and plant-based nutrition are two such medical breakthroughs.

Like other influential advancements in the history of medicine, these practices have, at times, been discounted or even completely rejected by "the system" due to a variety of reasons—money, government policies, long-held beliefs, and even egos and pride. It is not the first time this has happened in modern medicine and certainly won't be the last. I hope great things will prevail as did with the following two examples of scientific discoveries.

In the late 1840s Dr. Ignaz Semmelweis, a Hungarian obstetrician, made the simple observation that hand washing could dramatically reduce the spread of infectious diseases.[1] He had noticed this effect when a significant reduction in maternal deaths was seen between two adjacent birthing clinics.

As part of their normal duties, physicians in the first clinic were routinely transitioning between performing autopsies in the morgue and delivering babies in the maternity center. These physicians did not wash their hands between these tasks as this was not a standard of practice during that time. Infections and death affected an average of one of every ten women in this clinic.

In the second clinic, the midwives were also busy delivering babies but did not perform autopsies as part of their routine duties. The infection and death rates in this clinic were almost nonexistent and puzzled clinicians at the time. The resulting spread of deadly infectious bacteria in the first clinic from cadavers to young mothers was later discovered by Dr. Semmelweis and found to be directly due to the lack of hand washing. After he implemented a policy of hand washing between patients, the death rates plummeted in the first clinic and were in line with those of the second clinic.

The life-saving benefits of hand washing uncovered by Dr. Semmelweis during this time conflicted with the current scientific and medical opinions of his peers. As a result, Dr. Semmelweis was persecuted and even rejected by his colleagues for proposing such an outlandish theory. After lashing out at his critics for their judgmental views of his "radical" ideas on hand washing and proper hygiene, he was forced by others to enter a mental institution. They thought he was crazy! He later died at this institution due to septicemia caused by injuries sustained during a beating from the guards.

Dr. Semmelweis's work did not earn the respect it deserved until well after his death when the germ theory of disease was developed by Louis Pasteur in the 1870s, proving the exact same link between sanitization and the spread of infectious disease.

Another medical breakthrough initially dismissed by our current medical system was the discovery of *Helicobacter pylori* as the primary cause of gastritis and peptic ulcer disease. Ulcers were always thought to have been due to stress and lifestyle factors, which increased the acidity level in the stomach. Conventional treatment consisted of drinking milk and taking antacids. The problem with this approach was this: the ulcers never completely went away, turning this painful condition into a chronic disease or even cancer for some patients.

Enter onto the scene Drs. Barry Marshall and Robin Warren in 1982. They noticed spiral-shaped bacteria in the biopsies of patients with stomach ulcers. These two great minds had just discovered *H. pylori,* which we now know is responsible for 80 to 90 percent of all duodenal and gastric ulcers.[2]

At the time, many in the medical and scientific community, including gastroenterologists and bacteriologists, found this idea absurd! These practitioners thought the notion of curing ulcers simply by treating the *H. pylori* infection with a short-term course of antibiotics to be far too simplistic. They were even insulted by the very thought of this.

Drug companies also vehemently rejected the idea as they were making millions from highly profitable anti-ulcer drugs. In the ultimate form of experimentation Dr. Marshall deliberately infected himself by swallowing a suspension of colonized *H. pylori.* Within a matter of days he was experiencing bloating, fullness, bad breath, and vomiting.[3] An endoscopy showed severe gastritis proving the cause-and-effect relationship his colleagues had previously refused to accept.

It wasn't until nearly a decade later in 1991 that the Centers for Disease Control formally declared the link between *H. pylori* and gastric disease. In 2005, Marshall and Warren received the ultimate award for their extraordinary pioneering work—a Nobel Prize in Physiology or Medicine for their discovery of *H. pylori.*[4]

Shortfalls in the Current Medical Education System

In the six years I attended pharmacy school, I did not receive one single lecture on how nutrition affects the human body. This may not be surprising to you, especially in a society where drugs, and not food, are the most sought-after form of treatment.

What is surprising is the lack of nutritional training for doctors in medical school. One would think that if anyone, other than a registered dietitian, would need the knowledge on how nutrition affects a person's overall health status that this would be a physician. After all, they are the individuals best in position to help others fight through their illnesses and reclaim their health.

Sadly, nothing could be further from the truth. This statement isn't meant to discredit all the hard work physicians go through in order to get the knowledge and expertise they acquire in medical school. Doctors don't subject themselves to the rigors and demands of such programs if they aren't willing to dedicate their lives to the well-being of others. What is important to highlight, however, is the large shortfall or complete absence of any credible nutritional courses in our current medical education system. Unfortunately, doctors are being shortchanged by a system that focuses on drugs, surgeries, and procedures to fix everything.

More than twenty-five years ago the National Research Council identified deficiencies in the curricula of U.S. medical schools. Nutritional teachings were one of these deficiencies. The prestigious reviewers recommended that nutrition become a required course in every U.S. medical school, with a minimum of twenty-five hours of coursework devoted to this topic.[5]

Since then little progress has been made. In all actuality the situation has gotten worse. In the latest survey of medical schools released in 2010 only 25 percent of schools required even a single course on nutrition, down from 30 percent of schools in 2004.[6] Overall, medical students received an average of only 19.6 contact hours on nutrition, down from an average of 22.3 contact hours in 2004. This fails to meet the minimum recommended amount by the National Research Council and falls disastrously short of what's actually needed to make a meaningful difference in the lives of patients. And consider that doctors who attended medical school years before that may have never received any nutrition training (perhaps your own physician).

Recent data have shown a declining interest in the topic of nutrition by physicians despite studies showing the importance of targeted nutritional therapy in the reduction of morbidity (disease) and mortality (death).[7] Medical students are also following in physicians' footsteps as their perception of the importance of clinical nutritional knowledge decreases as they progress through medical school. This stands to reason since the deeper one gets into medical school, the more entrenched a person is with the depth of information offered about medications and surgeries being used as the only or primary source of treatment for patients.

These findings are disturbing, but what's more disturbing is the fact that patients sometimes know more than their doctors when tested on basic nutritional knowledge. The *American Journal of Clinical Nutrition* reported this fact when putting patients and physicians head-to-head in an exam on practical nutritional knowledge. They found that 52 percent of patients scored higher than the lowest score by a physician, and 7 percent of patients scored higher than the average physician on the exam.[8]

> **Patients sometimes know more than their doctors when tested on basic nutritional knowledge.**

Certainly there is a need for increasing the amount of nutrition education in medical schools. What's also needed is an emphasis on changing the mindset of current or soon-to-be medical doctors on the importance of this critical topic.

Efforts are being made to make this a reality, but these efforts share the same resistance as the two examples you read about in the beginning of this chapter. Resistance in the medical community, the mindset of the general public, activities of special interest groups, and actions of elected officials are all stacked against the case for proper instruction on nutrition in the medical community. A case in point can be seen in Dr. John McDougall's work.

Dr. McDougall is a medical doctor who has been using nutrition as the main course of therapy to treat and cure his patients of chronic diseases for over forty years. He drafted a bill introduced into the California legislature aimed at requiring some basic nutritional continuing education requirements for currently practicing physicians and surgeons.[9] When initially brought forward in February 2011 California Senate Bill 380 (SB 380) called for a one-time requirement of twelve hours of continuing education on the subject of nutrition and lifestyle behavior for the treatment of chronic diseases. Physicians with a California license would be given until December 31, 2016, to complete this requirement, giving them a little more than five years to do so.

The California Medical Association (CMA) wasn't fond of this requirement and didn't think their physicians should be mandated to participate in a one-time continuing education requirement on nutrition and health. They subsequently opposed this mandate in legislative hearings citing examples of other solutions currently being offered to bridge the gap on nutrition and health. These examples included soda companies putting the total number of calories on the front of their product labels and Michelle Obama's Let's Move! campaign. Any continuing education mandate, according to CMA, could lead to "unintended consequences" for their members.[10]

The California Orthopedic Association and the California Academy of Family Physicians also opposed any requirements in this bill for nutrition-related continuing education hours due to the time required and difficulty that would be experienced by their member physicians in meeting these requirements. These objections actually came after the bill had already been amended to require just seven hours of one-time continuing nutrition education credits instead of the original twelve hours.

In the end, SB 380 did pass but not after being further amended. The final result requires the California State Medical Board to "periodically disseminate information and educational material regarding the prevention and treatment of chronic disease by the application of changes in nutrition and lifestyle behavior."[11] In other words, the state medical board must mail a pamphlet or some reading material every once in a while to each licensed physician in California on the subject of nutrition.

Do you honestly think physicians will actually take the time to read this material and learn from it? Human nature doesn't always lend itself to a person voluntarily engaging in a specified activity unless there is a personal desire or passion to do so (or some financial reward). We can only hope that working in a profession that has everything to do with healing people would be reason enough to take an interest in this subject.

There is some good news on the forefront despite setbacks like these. A few organizations have noticed the need for high-quality formal training to be offered on the subject of nutrition and health. Courses are now being offered for both medical professionals and the general public to learn more about these topics. These courses are on a voluntary basis and include the following programs:

- Certificate Program in Plant-Based Nutrition, T. Colin Campbell Foundation and eCornell University (http://nutritionstudies.org)

- The Starch Solution Certification Course for Healthcare Professionals, John McDougall, MD (http://www.drmcdougall. com/health/programs/starch-solution-certification-course/)

- The Diet and Lifestyle Intervention Course, Wellness Forum Institute for Health Studies (http://www.wellnessforuminstitute. org/programs.html)

- The Nutrition Educator Diploma Program, Wellness Forum Institute for Health Studies (http://www.wellnessforuminstitute. org/programs.html)

- Food for Life Certification Program, Physicians Committee for Responsible Medicine (http://www.pcrm.org/health/diets/ffl/ training)

- Nutritional Education Trainer Certification Program (NETCP), Joel Fuhrman, MD (http://www.nutritionaleducation.com)

- Hippocrates Health Educator Program, Hippocrates Health Institute (http://hippocratesinst.org/health-educator-program)

Our medical education system may be failing to provide the education needed for physicians to take on the challenges we face in the twenty-first century, but this will only lead to opportunities for organizations and individuals like these to pick up the slack and offer solutions for those interested in viable alternatives.

Behind the Scenes of Medicine

Money, or the desire to accumulate wealth, has become just as entrenched into our cultural values as baseball and apple pie in America. Like it or not, we are programmed to think this way from the first time we earn a paycheck at our very first job. The vision of acquiring and spending money in order to live the American dream is everywhere you look these days, and it's no better executed than at the top where corporate and political interests align.

A lot of spending happening behind the scenes in today's political and social settings is done with only one motive in mind—to boost the profits of big business instead of improving the lives of average citizens. The health-care industry is no different from any other industry. It wants to produce as many profits as possible. This is one of the reasons why the safest, least costly, and most effective medical treatments (that is, plant-based nutrition and lifestyle medicine) are not being utilized like they should to combat the gluttony of chronic diseases seen today.

The ineffective allocation of our financial resources occurs in a variety of forms. It's important to understand why and how these things have come to be in order to understand why our current healthcare system works the way it does.

Propublica is an independent, nonprofit news agency that produces investigative journalism in the public interest. They publish and update the Dollars for Docs database (http://projects.propublica.org/docdollars) detailing payments made to doctors on behalf of different pharmaceutical companies including some of the more well-known big pharmas—Pfizer, Merck, GlaxoSmithKline, Eli Lilly, Johnson & Johnson, and AstraZeneca, among others.[12] These payments are made to doctors, pharmacists, medical institutions, and other healthcare providers for consulting services, speaking fees, research, business travel, meals, educational items and gifts, and royalty or license fees to promote awareness and sales of certain pharmaceutical drugs.

Over a four-year time span, from 2009 to 2012, Propublica reported a total of $2.1 billion dollars in payments from fifteen pharmaceutical companies being made to physicians, medical institutions, and other healthcare providers. Keep in mind this report does not include all payments from all drug companies since federal law has only legally required companies to report these data since 2014 as part of the Affordable Care Act.

What this report does do is provide transparency from the data currently available to show any relationships that may exist among medical professionals and pharmaceutical companies. Not all physicians receive direct payments, and it's important to point this out. It's also important for the general public to realize this information is available if they choose to do more research into it.

Pharmaceutical companies are quite persistent about getting their foot in the door of doctors' offices and hospitals to talk about their latest blockbuster drug. They often cater in all-expense-paid meals to doctors' offices (for all staff) or pass out invitations to attend free dinner events conducted at upscale restaurants where information is then presented about their new products.

> **Pharmaceutical companies are quite persistent about getting their foot in the door of doctors' offices.**

Early in my career I attended some of these functions, but now I sincerely regret it knowing they were limiting my perspective on available treatment options for several chronic illnesses at the expense of driving up overall healthcare costs. I realize now how the utilization of marketing dollars promotes what many times are ineffective medications in the continuation of sick care in this country instead of promoting safer, cost-free alternatives such as plant-based nutrition and lifestyle medicine. Because of this not-so-hidden motive behind lavish pharmaceutical-paid events, I no longer participate in them. I frequently tell others there's one thing you can count on me never eating—food supplied by a drug company regardless of how healthy it is.

You can see how the aforementioned examples can foster direct relationships between medical practitioners and pharmaceutical companies. Even though direct kickbacks for prescribing specific drugs is illegal, the money and gifts bestowed from drug companies to medical practitioners only serves to form a sort of "silent agreement" to favor the use of specific products and treatment options for certain diseases. This ultimately affects what forms of medical care are offered to the patient. These same phenomena happen in the world of politics and medicine but on a much larger scale. Truth be told, it acts to form the blueprint for how our healthcare system is currently set up to operate.

Lobbying and Healthcare

The Center for Responsive Politics keeps track of special interest and lobbying contributions and activities within American politics. According to their data, the health industry was the number one spender, more than any other industry, in terms of total lobbying contributions made from 1998 to 2011.[13]

The health industry spent just over $4.7 billion over this fourteen-year period, and the largest contributor within this industry was the pharmaceutical and health products sector. They spent a total of $2.27 billion or nearly half of all healthcare-related lobbying dollars. This works out to an average of $444,227 per day for this period spent by the drug and medical device companies to "butter up" their political allies. Individual contributors within the pharmaceutical and health products sector include many companies with household names such as Pfizer, Merck, Eli Lilly, and Johnson & Johnson, just to name a few.

In order to spend this kind of money, you have to have a lot of foot soldiers hitting the pavement for you. A total of 3,223 lobbyists were reportedly working for the health industry alone in 2010. This same year the U.S. Department of Health and Human Services had a total of 1,208 lobbyists vying for their attention.

These kinds of lobbying efforts and financial contributions do not fall on deaf ears. It only takes a quick look around America to see this. While the demand for prescription drugs and medical devices is going up, thanks to the lobbying efforts and dollars spent by pharmaceutical companies, our overall state of health is declining and so are our bank accounts. Over 62 percent of all bankruptcies reported in 2007 were due to medical debt, according to the *American Journal of Medicine*.[14]

Can you imagine how different our nation's landscape would be if the billions of dollars spent, directly or indirectly for ineffective medical care, were instead allocated to methods that actually worked? There will always be a need for medications and surgeries as long as infectious diseases, acute traumatic events, and other rare medical conditions occur, but twenty-first-century medicine is dealing with a different monster. This monster isn't responding to more pills and procedures. It's responding to eating a healthy supply of plant-based, whole foods and engaging in regular exercise.

The Effect of Big Agriculture on the Health of a Nation

Our government provides billions of dollars in food subsidies to the agricultural industry every year. These subsidies play a major role in determining which foods are grown and in what quantities they're grown on farms across America. Farmers will typically grow whatever crops generate the highest amount of income for their efforts. Since the output of American farms is determined largely by what crops are subsidized, it's safe to say these subsidies invariably dictate which foods end up on the plates of millions of Americans at the end of the day. Unfortunately, animal-based and processed foods are the foods most often claiming these spots.

The U.S. Department of Agriculture (USDA) has been keeping track of what America eats since 1909.[15] From 1909 to 2007 there has been a dramatic increase in the annual consumption of the following foods:

- Meat intake went from 123.9 pounds to 200.6 pounds per year per person
- Cheese consumption increased eightfold from 3.8 pounds to 31.4 pounds per year per person
- Use of oils more than doubled from 35.4 pounds to 86.7 pounds per year per person
- Use of sweeteners increased from 119 pounds to 136.4 pounds per year per person
- Frozen dairy consumption went from 1.5 pounds to 25.3 pounds per year per person

The increased availability of low-nutrient, inexpensive foods containing high amounts of fat and sugar, similar to those just mentioned, along with refined grains are the main contributors to the rise in obesity and decline in public health seen in the United States in recent decades.[16]

If we are to tackle these problems effectively, then it is imperative we approach them at their most fundamental level—the utilization and output of American farmland. To do this we must understand how our tax dollars and other available moneys flow through the system. Then we need to find ways to improve this.

From 1995 to 2010 the USDA gave out a total of $261.9 billion in subsidies.[17] The top 10 percent of farm program recipients received 74 percent of the total subsidies. This works out to an average of $30,751 per year for each of these recipients. Smaller-scale farming operations only received an average of $587 per year per recipient. This means smaller, independent farmers trying to make a living are literally left to fend for themselves while large corporate operations make out like kings.

In addition, 64 percent of these subsidies supported the production of commodity crops. The five most heavily subsidized commodity crops were corn, wheat, cotton, soybeans, and rice. The vast majority of these commodity crops were used for animal feed instead of being consumed directly by humans. The Institute for Agriculture and Trade Policy reported in 2006 that 60 percent of all corn and 47 percent of all soy produced in the U.S. was used as feed for domestic livestock production.[18]

The use of a majority of these subsidy programs promotes the production of foods that are contributing to serious illnesses in our country. Dairy products are an example. The dairy industry has subsidy programs set up to ensure their continued use and profitability. The Milk Income Loss Contract (MILC) program protects dairy producers by providing direct payments to producers when the average price of milk drops below a minimum level.[19] Another program called the Dairy Product Price Support Program allows the USDA to set a minimum price for nonfat dry milk, butter, and cheese. Under this program the USDA will buy any excess dairy products from producers and store these excess products in warehouses until the products are sold or donated.[20] Both of these programs help protect dairy producers from losing money while encouraging excess production of their products. They're essentially slush funds.

Livestock producers also benefit from an array of subsidy programs. These programs provide marketing support along with emergency funds and price supports. They include the Livestock Compensation Program, Emergency Livestock Feed Assistance Program, and the Livestock Emergency Assistance Program.[21] In addition to these programs, the Environmental Quality Incentives Program helps livestock producers reduce their production costs by providing funding to clean up pollution and reduce soil erosion caused by their operations in the first place.[22]

Fruit and vegetable farmers are not this lucky. These health-promoting foods are considered "specialty crops" by the USDA. Specialty crops are disqualified from receiving any direct subsidies. The only form of subsidy support for these crops comes in the form of subsidized crop insurance, which helps compensate producers for losses due to weather or natural disasters.[23] Furthermore, the government forbids farmers who participate in commodity subsidy programs, which produce cheap corn and soy for animal feed, from growing fruits and vegetables on their land. This arrangement puts our nation's farmers who wish to grow healthy, sustainable food at a disadvantage by encouraging them to produce commodity crops instead of fresh fruits and vegetables with higher rates of return. Essentially, your tax dollars are funding disease and sickness as an end result.

Lobbying and Agriculture

The lobbying activities on behalf of special interest groups toward the USDA paints a clear picture as to why the subsidy programs are the way they are. In 2010 alone, the USDA had a total of 943 lobbyists vying for their attention.[24] Individual companies with lobbyists working on their behalf include the following: National Milk Producers Federation, National Pork Producers Council, Monsanto, Kraft Foods, Nestle SA, Cargill Inc., Smithfield Foods, Dean Foods, Tyson Foods, and the McDonald's Corp.

Here is a description of the products and services provided by just a few of these companies:

- Tyson Foods is one of the world's largest processors and marketers of chicken, beef, and pork.
- Smithfield Foods is the world's largest producer and processor of pork.
- Dean Foods is the largest U.S. processor and distributor of milk, creamer, and cultured dairy products.
- Cargill is a major provider of animal feed and also one of the largest meat processing companies in the U.S.
- Monsanto is the world's largest producer of the herbicide glyphosate found in Roundup (weed killer) and the largest producer of genetically engineered seeds in the U.S.

Unfortunately, there is no National Kale Council, National Blueberry Federation, or Cruciferous Vegetable Producers Organization. The game of who can spend the most money on Capitol Hill is a one-sided affair when it comes to handing out lobbying contributions.

Millions of dollars have been spent over the years to ensure continued subsidy support from the USDA for the meat and dairy industries. Over a fourteen-year timespan, from 1998 to 2011, the livestock, dairy, egg, and poultry industries have spent approximately $98.4 million on lobbying efforts. This money not only bolsters support for subsidies but also helps to assure the USDA continues to write dietary guidelines favoring the consumption of these same products.

As a result, a major conflict of interest develops since we have the same government agency who is responsible for both the development of "healthy" dietary guidelines and for the promotion of our nation's agriculture production of inexpensive and unhealthy foods.

Perhaps it's time to give the responsibility for developing the U.S. dietary guidelines and food subsidy programs to an entity more in touch with the current state of disease and sickness going on in America. The Centers for Disease Control and Prevention would fit this role quite nicely. Their mission statement echoes these intentions: "To collaborate to create the expertise, information, and tools that people and communities need to protect their health—through health promotion, prevention of disease, injury and disability, and preparedness for new health threats."[25]

Contrast the CDC's mission with that of the USDA: "We provide leadership on food, agriculture, natural resources, and related issues based on sound public policy, the best available science, and efficient management."[26] As it stands, the word *health* is mentioned three times in the CDC's statement but not a single time in the USDA's mission.

The only way we're going to change the system is to change the way we spend our money. Every time you as an individual spend money on a product or service, whether it be fast food, a pharmaceutical drug, or ineffective medical care, you are supporting those industries. When you change your buying habits to support everyday healthy living by adopting a whole foods, plant-based lifestyle, you not only reap the rewards in terms of better overall health, but also lower the demand for the continuation of our current system of counterintuitive agricultural practices and dysfunctional medical care.

It's a win-win situation for you as an individual and for your average citizen. Everyone gets healthy. We all lead more productive lives. Our economy becomes stronger and more financially stable over time due to the reduction in spending on healthcare and increased productivity as a nation. This makes us more competitive on a global scale. There's really no good reason not to take these steps. The best part about all this: you can do something starting right now. You don't have to wait for the rich and powerful to change "the system" in order for you to start eating well and exercising. You just have to start.

Part II

The Food for Health Program

A Healthful New Menu

"No single food will make or break good health.
But the kinds of food you choose day in and day
out have a major impact."

—WALTER WILLET, MD

Every day a new diet program is popping up claiming to be the end-all cure all. You're constantly bombarded with television infomercials, radio ads, pamphlets, magazine articles, billboards, and "friends" touting plans and programs and diet pills and gimmicks of all kinds. With all this information thrown your way, it's easy to become confused about nutrition and health.

You may be asking yourself, *Should I follow a low-carb or high-protein diet? Is low-fat dairy or dairy-free the way to go? Which is better the Mediterranean Diet, Atkins Diet, or Paleo Diet? How about Weight Watchers or The Zone?* It's almost inevitable that most people will fail time after time on various programs and fad diets. This is great news for the companies because they continue to get repeat business as customers hand over their hard-earned dollars for ineffective approaches.

Dieting shouldn't be this difficult and it doesn't have to be. In order to set the record straight, I want you to do something that might sound counterintuitive, if not a bit crazy. Ready? Throw the dieting word right out the window! Get rid of it, forever.

Dieting doesn't work because it only focuses on short-term results instead of long-term success. I'm going to outline for you a much simpler and more understandable way of eating. This new way of eating works. It works because it focuses on making lifestyle changes instead of engaging in the yo-yo effect of on-again off-again dieting programs.

> Dieting doesn't work because it only focuses on short-term results instead of long-term success.

I'm going to help you develop a basic understanding of which foods promote health and which foods promote disease. This will empower you to make better choices every single time you pick up your fork, knife, and spoon. The same foods that promote health also tend to promote weight loss, while the foods that promote disease tend to promote weight gain. By gaining an understanding of these simple concepts, you'll learn how different foods affect the human body and be able to skip the diets altogether. You can then develop a healthful way of eating tailored to your unique tastes and turn these new meals into an everyday habit and lifelong journey of prospering health. Let's get started.

Adopting the *Food For Health* Lifestyle

My *Food For Health* eating guide is comprised of two simple principles to help you achieve both maximum weight loss and optimal health. These two principles consist of learning which foods to include in your daily menu and which foods to avoid. This eating plan provides a powerful new foundation aimed to assist you in your health-centered journey. I encourage you to refer to this guide anytime you need to.

As you can see, it's important to incorporate a variety of whole foods from the plant kingdom—vegetables, fruits, legumes, whole grains, and nuts and seeds—in order to get maximum results. These foods are beneficial because they are generally low in fat, contain no cholesterol, have an abundance of fiber, and contain thousands of powerful phytonutrients and antioxidants needed to fight chronic diseases.

In contrast, foods that should be avoided or eliminated—meat, dairy, eggs, processed foods, and refined carbs/sugars—are typically high in fat,

Food FoRx Health Guide©

Include   Avoid

Vegetables
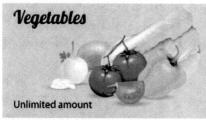
Unlimited amount

Meat
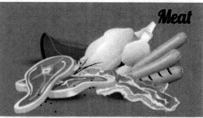

Fruits
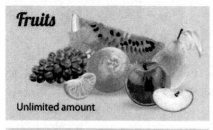
Unlimited amount

Dairy
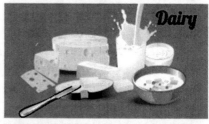

Legumes
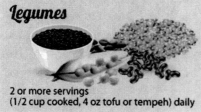
2 or more servings
(1/2 cup cooked, 4 oz tofu or tempeh) daily

Eggs
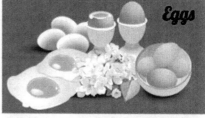

Whole Grains
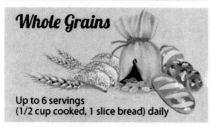
Up to 6 servings
(1/2 cup cooked, 1 slice bread) daily

Processed Foods
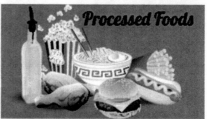

Nuts & Seeds
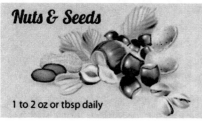
1 to 2 oz or tbsp daily

Refined Carbs or Sugars
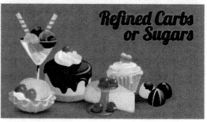

high in cholesterol, contain little or no fiber, and completely lack any phytonutrients essential to achieving optimal health.

This new eating style may come as a bit of a shock to you. If you feel a deep sense of uneasiness about this unfamiliar lifestyle, then don't worry. It's okay to feel this way. I, too, had great apprehension about making such profound changes in my everyday food selections before switching to this new lifestyle. Let this information sink in a bit. Don't worry about being deemed a failure if you don't immediately empty out your refrigerator, restock it with organically grown alfalfa sprouts, and become the next poster child for the centenarian club. That's not what this is about, nor is it about converting you into a vegetarian or vegan as part of some ulterior motive. After all, you could follow a vegan diet comprised of French fries, Fruit Loops®, and soda pop and end up morbidly obese and unhealthy. That's not what I want for you.

Instead, my *Food For Health* guide is aimed at empowering you to become the best you can be, living a life free of disease for years to come. Your future doesn't have to include a heart attack, stroke, or diabetes. Nor does it have to include future financial hardships due to a never-ending stack of prescription co-pays and medical bills. With this new knowledge and a commitment to following my *Food For Health* lifestyle, you'll see results within a few short weeks. Your energy levels will begin to rise and your body will start to transform into a much healthier version of you. This is exactly what Bev experienced in her transformation.

Bev's Story

Bev grew up her entire life following what many would consider a healthy lifestyle. She was active, ate plenty of fruits and vegetables, and consumed lean meats for protein. She and her family had always done their best to stay away from fast foods and fried foods. She was very much concerned about the high amount of fat found in these foods and the effect this would have on her overall health. Her husband had worked most of his career as a pharmacist, and they both were diligent about taking their daily vitamins along with a few other supplements when they got sick.

Bev remained slim and enjoyed the benefits of this lifestyle until her early fifties. At that time, she started gaining weight and her blood pressure and cholesterol levels started creeping up. It wasn't long before her blood sugars soared out of control too leading to a diagnosis of type 2 diabetes. She would consistently see blood glucose levels as high as 180–200 mg/dl.

Over the next two decades her diabetes continued to get worse. At the same time, she proceeded to experience high blood pressure problems. Her readings often exceeded 160/80 putting her in the high-risk category. Her cholesterol levels were also dangerously elevated. Bev's total cholesterol topped out at over 280 mg/dl and her LDL cholesterol was over 190 mg/dl. She was a heart attack waiting to happen! This all despite taking numerous medications to try and control the barrage of warning signs of her chronic illnesses.

On a summer day in June 2005, Bev temporarily lost vision in one eye while experiencing pain down her arm. She was rushed to the emergency room by her husband. No initial heart attack was diagnosed; however, Bev failed a stress test and was sent for an angiogram the next morning to look inside the blood vessels surrounding her heart. The doctors found a total of eight blockages, many occluded over 90 percent of the affected coronary arteries.

Bev underwent major open heart surgery as doctors performed multiple bypasses in hopes of repairing her damaged heart. When she left the hospital, she was taking over ten medications for her heart disease and diabetes. The number of medications would've been higher had she not failed previous therapy with numerous cholesterol-lowering drugs, including statin drugs, which caused undesirable side effects.

Despite these medical interventions, she returned only five months after undergoing open heart surgery to have a stent placed in one of the major arteries leading to her kidneys. The blockages just wouldn't go away. Bev was now experiencing the beginning stages of kidney failure. Over the next four years her health would continue to deteriorate. She eventually reached stage four kidney disease. If not halted, this condition would lead to the complete failure of both her kidneys. The only option at that point would be an unlikely bid for a kidney transplant or lifelong dialysis.

Bev was now 40 pounds overweight and suffered from an assortment of chronic diseases—coronary artery disease, type 2 diabetes, high cholesterol, high blood pressure, irritable bowel syndrome, arthritis, kidney disease, diabetic retinopathy, and sleep apnea. She was also constantly fighting off frequent upper respiratory and sinus infections due to a weakened immune system.

If that weren't enough, she had to go in every three months for laser treatments on her eyes to fend off possible blindness as a result of her diabetes. To top it off, her gastroenterologist had now found precancerous polyps in her colon. Bev felt absolutely hopeless at this point and desperately prayed for answers as her ailing body continued to go downhill.

Her prayers were finally answered in 2009 when her gastroenterologist informed her about the Complete Health Improvement Program (CHIP). CHIP is a program designed to help individuals achieve an optimal state of health by promoting a whole foods, plant-based lifestyle. Bev immediately jumped on board. This opportunity was her second chance at life, and she began to learn about the benefits of plant-based nutrition right away.

She made significant changes to her diet, consuming nothing but plant-based, whole foods while at the same time eliminating her familiar Standard American Diet. Bev continues to eat this way today while rarely consuming animal-based or processed foods, approximately only once or twice a month, if that.

Two years into the program, Bev is a brand new youthful seventy-eight years old. She states she's a completely new person and is convinced she'll live a better quality of life, if not longer life, after switching to this plant-based lifestyle. She has chosen to take back control of her own health and continues to see improvement every single day. Her diabetes has dramatically improved as her blood sugars are consistently in the normal range despite getting rid of all but one oral diabetic medication. She's nearly eliminated the need for any insulin shots as well, using as little as 0–2 units of Novolog insulin per meal. That's a remarkable turnaround for a woman who used to inject herself with 65 units of insulin a day while still seeing blood sugar levels hovering over 200 mg/dl.

Bev's heart disease has also started to reverse. Her total cholesterol dropped over 93 points and her LDL cholesterol dropped over 101 points since beginning the CHIP program. Her blood pressure readings are back to normal despite lowering the doses of half of her blood pressure medications by 50 percent. She continues to have discussions with her physician about further dosage reductions as her condition improves.

In addition, many of Bev's other medical conditions have completely reversed or dramatically improved. She's lost over 40 pounds and no longer has any signs of arthritis, sleep apnea, or irritable bowel syndrome. She also hasn't experienced an upper respiratory infection in over two years since adopting a whole foods, plant-based lifestyle. Her vision has improved and her diabetic retinopathy has completely gone away with no further requirements for expensive laser eye treatments. Best of all, her kidney disease has started to reverse. She's no longer facing the prospect of losing her kidneys and having to go on dialysis for the rest of her life.

Bev is living proof that it's never too late to turn your life (and your health) around. Her power-packed menu of plant-based, whole foods has accomplished in two years what modern medicine failed to do in twenty-five years for her—restore her body's ability to heal itself despite the damage that's already been done to it.

Consume a Variety of Plant-Based, Whole Foods

My *Food For Health* guide consists of five categories of foods essential for healthy living. These five building blocks provide an abundance of flavor and variety. With the following foods you can make simple, delicious recipes such as cinnamon walnut oatmeal, spicy garden chili, black bean and brown rice burgers, or hot apple crisp. The choices are endless and boredom is not in the plant-based vocabulary.

Vegetable Group

This category of food contains some of the most nutrient-dense foods on the face of the planet because it is also the healthiest food group to eat from. Vegetables are naturally low in fat, high in potassium, and contain no cholesterol resulting in lower blood pressure readings, reduced risks of heart disease and diabetes, and lower rates of osteoporosis and kidney disease.[1]

The various colors contained within the vegetable group provide clues to their powerful nutritional benefits. For example, orange vegetables such as carrots and pumpkins are loaded with beta-carotene essential for healthy eyes and cancer protection. Green veggies are high in calcium for strong bones and folate to support optimal brain health. Lycopene found in red bell peppers and tomatoes helps support heart health and acts as a potent cancer-fighting agent. All these vibrant colors are nature's way of displaying the life-giving properties the plant kingdom has to offer.

The following chart displays the nutrient density of different vegetables to help you understand which ones pack the most power to their punch in terms of their ability to promote optimal health. Dark leafy greens lead the way at the top of the list, but it's important to include as many vegetables as you can in your daily menu in whatever manner works best for you.

Feel free to enjoy an unlimited amount of servings from this group each day. It is impossible to overdose on vegetables. The more you eat, the more it opens up your taste buds to this wonderful group of foods. You'll be surprised at how delicious vegetables really can be.

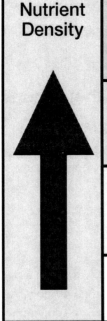

Nutrient Density	**Dark Leafy Greens** Kale, mustard greens, collard greens, arugula, romaine lettuce, watercress, dandelion greens, turnip greens, spinach, swiss chard, bok choy, parsley
	Cruciferous Vegetables (Non-leafy green varieties) Broccoli, brussels sprouts, cauliflower, turnips, radishes, cabbage
	Non-Starchy Vegetables Bell peppers, asparagus, celery, okra, garlic, zucchini, tomatoes, mushrooms, artichoke, onions, cucumbers, string beans, eggplant
	Starchy Vegetables Potatoes, sweet potato, corn, yams, pumpkins, squash, parsnips

Data Source: *Eat For Health* by Joel Fuhrman, M.D.

Fruit Group

An apple a day really can keep the doctor away. In fact, eating five or more items of fruit per day has been shown to decrease the risk of coronary heart disease by 60 percent.[2] Statin drugs, by contrast, only boast of a slightly less than 30 percent reduction in coronary events and are often accompanied by an array of side effects—muscle pain and weakness, memory loss, nausea, gas, abdominal cramping, flushing, increased blood sugar levels, and even liver damage.[3]

Although many people believe that eating too much fruit is a bad thing because of the sugar content, this is not the case. Nearly all fruits are lower on the glycemic index, meaning they do not cause a rapid spike in blood sugars. They're also packed full of antioxidants and phytonutrients making them an excellent choice as part of a healthy diet.

Berries, in particular, are rich in compounds called anthocyanins responsible for the dark shades of red, purple, and blue found in familiar fruits such as blueberries, strawberries, blackberries, and raspberries. Berries are one of the best fruits to eat and are widely known for their ability to improve cardiovascular health, reduce age-induced oxidative stress, and prevent a number of degenerative diseases.[4]

In addition to berries, feel free to include as many fresh and frozen fruits as possible in your diet. Buy fruit that isn't packaged with any added sugar to ensure getting the maximum health benefits from this group. Choose from an array of low-fat, tasty treats in the form of apples, pears, bananas, oranges, grapes, melons, kiwi, mangoes, grapefruit, peaches, apricots, cherries, pineapple, and more. You simply can't go wrong when consuming nature's sweetest gifts.

Legume Group

This group includes all varieties of beans, peas, lentils, and soy products. Legumes are commonly used in cultures throughout the world where low rates of obesity and chronic diseases are the norm. Unfortunately, they play only a minor role in diets of Westernized cultures where these diseases are now a growing epidemic.

Legumes are naturally low in fat, serve as an excellent source of dietary fiber, and provide ample amounts of protein (about 20–30 percent of their total calories). They are also high in essential nutrients such as folate, zinc, calcium, and iron. Whether you're indulging in a delicious hummus dip made from chickpeas or enjoying a bowl of black beans with brown rice, be sure to include the legume family as part of your regular menu.

Aim to get a minimum of two servings per day from this group. This equates to about one cup of cooked legumes. Feel free to eat more if you desire. Beans and lentils can also be consumed in their sprouted forms, which results in higher amounts of protein and other available nutrients versus their cooked forms.[5]

Legumes have been studied for numerous health benefits including their ability to lower cholesterol levels and maintain healthy blood sugars in both diabetic and nondiabetic individuals.[6] They play a role in the prevention and treatment of osteoporosis and heart disease and have been found to relieve menopausal symptoms in women.[7] Unprocessed or minimally processed soy foods such as edamame, tempeh, and tofu have been shown to decrease the risk of prostate, breast, and colorectal cancers.[8-10]

Whole Grain Group

The whole grain group consists of several food items including, but not limited to, brown rice, oats, barley, wheat, millet, rye, amaranth, quinoa, bulgur, spelt, kamut, and buckwheat. Cereals, breads, and pastas made from 100 percent whole grains are included in this category as well. Whole grains are a good source of complex carbohydrates, fiber, protein, and B vitamins. For those with a gluten-related disorder it's best to stay away from wheat, barley, rye, and other gluten-containing products. Experiment with different recipes using these ingredients and find the ones that work best for you.

Those who adopt a whole foods, plant-based lifestyle can tend to overdo it with the whole grain group and consume a majority of their calories from these foods. While whole grains are a healthy option, they're not as nutrient dense as vegetables, fruits, or legumes, so make sure a majority of your calories are coming from these first three groups. Ideally, no more than a third of daily calories should come from the whole grain group. You can still reap the rewards of improved weight management, lower the incidence of cardiovascular disease and diabetes, and improve overall digestive health.[11]

Nuts and Seeds

Nuts and seeds are an excellent way to obtain beneficial sources of essential fats. Western diets are dominated by "bad" fats—trans fats, saturated fats, and excessive amounts of omega-6 fatty acids. These all increase the risk of obesity, heart disease, and diabetes when consumed in high amounts.

Nuts and seeds, by contrast, are higher in the "good" fats. In particular, they're an ideal way to obtain heart-healthy omega-3 fatty acids. These essential fats must be obtained in your diet because the body cannot produce them on its own. Walnuts, hemp seeds, chia seeds, and ground flaxseeds are all excellent sources of omega-3 fatty acids.

Consuming foods that are rich in omega-3 fatty acids (including dark leafy greens, flaxseed, and walnuts) has been shown to aid in the secondary prevention of high blood pressure, coronary heart disease, type 2 diabetes, and a number of different autoimmune disorders.[12]

Nuts and seeds are also great sources of protein, fiber, iron, calcium, potassium, manganese, magnesium, copper, zinc, and vitamin E. In addition, flaxseeds are known for their high content of lignans. Lignans have been shown to provide protective effects against both breast and colon cancer.[13,14]

Including raw, unsalted nuts and seeds as part of a healthy diet is something you may want to consider. Small amounts of nuts and seeds are all that is needed in order to receive their benefits. It is important to understand that nuts and seeds are calorically-dense foods, meaning they're packed with large amounts of calories despite their small size. Approximately 70 to 90 percent of total calories in nuts and seeds come in the form of fat, so a little goes a long way.

Some individuals may be more sensitive than others to this fat content. Consequently, these people may find it hard to reach their ideal body weight by eating nuts and seeds. Leaving nuts and seeds out of their diet may work best for them. As a general rule, though, most people can afford to consume 1 to 2 ounces of nuts and seeds per day. This is equivalent to approximately one small handful or a half cup.

Try a variety of ways to incorporate nuts and seeds into your diet. You can add them to salads or desserts, make homemade dressings or dips, or top off a bowl of old-fashioned oats in the morning with them. The key is to use them as condiments to your meals and not consume them by the bagful. Also, some individuals may be allergic to nuts. Avoiding them is the only way to prevent any adverse effects that result from these allergies.

The Fabulous Five

You've just been introduced to five new fabulous food groups. These five food groups are your ticket to an incredible journey of extraordinary health. The more you incorporate these foods into your daily eating habits, the more results you'll see. For best results, try to obtain *all* of your calories from these five food groups. If this seems out of reach for you, then just do your best to start with them and build from there.

You'll begin to see significant improvements in your overall health and be able to minimize your risk of chronic diseases by adopting a plant-based lifestyle with at least 90 percent of your calories coming from the five food groups discussed in this chapter. This would be the equivalent of eating no more than two to three meals per week from the standard American cuisine of animal-based and processed foods. The remainder of your meals should come from plant-based, whole foods.

The Facts on Animal-Based and Processed Food

"The doctor of the future will give no medicines, but
will interest his patients in the care of the human frame,
in diet, and in the causes and prevention of disease."
—THOMAS EDISON

The second part of my *Food For Health* eating guide outlines foods that should be avoided or eliminated altogether as part of a healthy diet. This would include all animal-based and processed foods because these foods are the root cause of most debilitating, chronic diseases.

Heart disease, obesity, type 2 diabetes, and a host of other chronic illnesses rarely existed until modern times when animal-based and processed foods started covering the majority of our dinner plates. While many factors such as physical activity, smoking, alcohol use, stress, sleeping habits, and genetic predisposition play a factor in determining whether or not we succumb to these diseases, diet, by far, is the greatest predictor in deciding our fate. You are not doomed solely based on your genes. The foods you eat or don't eat will most likely determine the state of your long-term health and quality of life. A more in-depth look at this topic will give a much clearer picture of why this is so.

Avoid Animal-Based and Processed Foods

Full of Fat

One major reason for avoiding these foods is their fat content. Animal-based foods such as meat and dairy and processed foods such as French fries and potato chips often contain two to ten times more fat than healthy, plant-based foods. Much of this is in the form of trans fat or saturated fat, which is the worst kind of fat. These types of fats are converted by the liver into cholesterol leading to elevated levels of both total and LDL "bad" cholesterol in the body.[1] These increases in cholesterol are responsible for the formation of atherosclerotic plaques inside the walls of the blood vessels, which results in higher rates of angina (chest pain), coronary heart disease, heart attack, and stroke.[2]

The cardiovascular system isn't the only victim. High intakes of total fat, saturated fat, and cholesterol lead to cognitive decline and increase the risk of dementia as individuals get older.[3] The risk of developing type 2 diabetes also increases with a higher consumption of trans and saturated fat.[4]

The chart on the next page puts in perspective the different degrees of fat and cholesterol content in various foods. Notice that *all* animal foods contain cholesterol, and *no* plant foods contain cholesterol. Cholesterol is part of animal cell membranes; whereas, plant cell membranes are not comprised of measurable amounts of cholesterol.[5]

"Heart-Healthy" Oils Aren't So Healthy

One of the most misunderstood and harmful sources of fat in the diet comes from oils. All oils, including vegetable oils, contain 120 calories per tablespoon with 100 percent of these coming from fat. Oils include olive and canola oil, which are touted to be "heart healthy." They are not.

Many in the medical and scientific world, along with those in the food industry, lead you to believe these oils are healthy based on poor interpretation of the data. When various studies are analyzed, it's quite clear that the "benefits" of oils are not because people added olive oil to their diet, but rather because they replaced other items such as butter, margarine, or corn oil (which contain higher amounts of saturated fat) with olive oil rich in monounsaturated fat.[6] This form of substitution may reduce the incidence of cardiovascular disease, but it falls far short of eliminating risk entirely.

Fat and Cholesterol Content of Various Foods

Animal-Based and Processed Foods	Fat (% of Calories)	Cholesterol (mg)	Plant-Based Foods	Fat (% of Calories)	Cholesterol (mg)
Beef, ground, 90% lean	51	65	Sweet potato, baked	1	0
Chicken, skinless, light meat	28	47	Apple	3	0
Turkey, ground	50	79	Broccoli	9	0
Pork, ham, lean	35	52	Brown rice, long grained	7	0
Salmon (silver), Alaskan	36	58	Black beans	4	0
Cheese, cheddar	72	105	Pita bread, whole wheat	8	0
2% Milk	36	8	Rice milk, original	17	0
Potato chips, plain, unsalted	57	0	Strawberries	9	0
Granola bar, soft, plain	33	1	Tomato	11	0
Frozen yogurt, vanilla	31	2	Chickpeas (garbanzo beans)	13	0

*All servings sizes equal to 100 grams
Source: USDA National Nutrient Database for Standard Reference via www.NutritionData.com, Accessed August 27, 2011

In 2000, a study in the *Journal of the American College of Cardiology* examined the effects of the Mediterranean Diet and olive oil on blood flow. Researchers found that blood flow was reduced by 31 percent three hours after a meal rich in olive oil.[7] This was due to the acute damage done to the endothelial lining of blood vessel walls. Researchers concluded the beneficial components of a Mediterranean Diet didn't come from olive oil but rather from antioxidant-rich foods such as fruits and vegetables.

Another notable study compared the rates of ischemic heart disease (in other words, coronary heart disease) and fat-related cancers among the Mediterranean, Japanese, and American diets.[8] Japanese diets have an abundance of plant-based foods and include very limited amounts of fats and oils while Mediterranean diets contain a significant amount of calories in the form of fat from olive oil. The American diet derives most of its fat from meat, milk, and cheese.

Results of the study showed rates of ischemic heart disease two and a half times greater in the Mediterranean group and nearly five times greater in the American group than those of the Japanese. Fat-related cancers of the prostate, breast, uterus, and ovaries all increased significantly as participants went from the Japanese to the Mediterranean to the American diet. Heart disease and cancer are the top two killers in the industrialized world. This study proves just how important it is to adhere to a menu of low-fat, plant-based whole foods in order to avoid these killer diseases.

Olive oil contains approximately 87 percent of its calories from saturated and monounsaturated fats, both of which are nonessential fats the human body is capable of making on its own. It does, however, provide some essential fats in the form of omega-6 and omega-3 fatty acids. While omega-6 fatty acids are considered essential, they're also pro-inflammatory and when consumed in high amounts can be detrimental to overall health. Omega-3 fatty acids, on the other hand, have potent anti-inflammatory effects providing for a wide range of health benefits.

Consuming an ideal mix of omega-6 to omega-3 fatty acids in a ratio of 2:1 or 1:1 as part of a healthy diet has been shown to reduce the risk of developing a number of chronic diseases including cardiovascular disease.[9] Olive oil has a ratio of O6:O3 of nearly 13:1, far from healthy. This is even worse than what's found in an order of McDonald's French fries, which have a ratio of O6:O3 of just under 12:1.

You're not doing yourself a favor by consuming olive oil. You will not be protecting yourself from heart disease if you choose to do so. To achieve optimal health your best bet is to avoid all oils and to stay away from foods prepared, cooked, or fried with oils of any kind.

Dark Side of Dairy

Dairy has been promoted as an important source of calcium to build strong, healthy bones. There's more than meets the eye behind those milk mustaches of the *Got Milk?* commercials though. Although the dairy industry wants everyone to believe consuming their products promotes healthy growth and development, the exact opposite holds true.

Dairy products contain proteins that are much different than our proteins. This makes sense since a cow doesn't resemble a human and neither does their DNA or amino acid sequences. Unfortunately, this can lead to problems when humans drink another species' milk, which is exactly the case for children genetically predisposed to type 1 diabetes. When these infants and young children drink cow's milk, they are prone to an autoimmune response taking place against the foreign proteins found in cow's milk.[10] These foreign proteins share a resemblance to the beta cells found in the pancreas.

Consequently, the body's immune system ends up attacking its own pancreas cells rendering them useless and unable to produce insulin. This is the underlying cause of type 1 diabetes for some and why we're seeing higher rates of insulin-dependent diabetes in children.[11] The damage done to the pancreas is permanent, so kids affected by this will have to take insulin shots for the rest of their life.

Another major problem with dairy is the component casein—the main protein found in milk, cheese, yogurt, and other dairy products. Casein has been studied extensively over the years for its effect on human health especially relating to cancer, which I discussed in depth in chapter 5. What's been uncovered is surprising. A strong correlation between the progression of cancerous tumors and casein has surfaced on multiple occasions in numerous animal studies.[12,13]

The correlation between dairy and cancer progression also holds true in the real world for people. A study spanning a total of sixty-five years was conducted in Europe assessing dairy consumption and cancer risk in nearly 5,000 people. Investigators found that those who consumed the most dairy early in life had nearly three times the risk of developing colorectal cancer.[14] Colorectal cancer is the third most common cancer in the United States among both men and women.

Dairy also increases levels of a hormone called insulin-like growth factor 1 (IGF-1). This is concerning because increased levels of IGF-1 have been shown in several studies to increase the rates of hormone-related cancers, such as cancers of the breast, prostate, and ovaries.[15,16] It's also partially responsible for the development of acne in much of our younger generation.[17]

Hormones have their role in maintaining optimal health, but when IGF-1 is artificially increased due to dairy consumption, it creates serious health problems. Many of us are completely unaware of this because of the marketing efforts of the dairy industry to falsely promote the "benefits" of their products. Unfortunately, hundreds of thousands of people die unnecessarily from cancers that didn't have to happen because of dairy consumption.

These same advertising tactics are used to convince us that dairy is critical in building strong, healthy bones. This concept, in theory, should lead to less bone fractures the more that dairy is consumed. That's not the case. Hip fractures are a key marker used to predict the incidence of osteoporosis throughout the world. The data show that countries who consume the highest amounts of milk—Norway, Sweden, United States, Australia, and United Kingdom—have the highest rates of hip fractures throughout the world.[18,19] In contrast, regions consuming the lowest amounts of milk—Africa, China, Mexico, and Iran—have the lowest rates of hip fractures. How can that be?

The topic of bone health and osteoporosis consists of multiple factors and is very complex. It was once theorized that dairy consumption produced an acidic effect on the human body, which it does. This acidic effect would then have to be neutralized by pulling calcium out of the bones, thereby returning the body to its preferred state of alkalinity. This is not completely true, however. Recent data in the last decade have shown this hypothesis to have little, if any, validity when it comes to dairy having a negative effect on calcium loss from bone and overall bone health.[20]

Having said that, new data are out which may explain the role of dairy in being a contributing factor to osteoporosis. Studies now indicate that consumption of dairy products (especially cheese), along with meats and other processed foods, lead to excess intakes of dietary phosphorus.[21,22] This can disrupt hormonal regulation of phosphate, calcium, and vitamin D in the body, resulting in tissue damage and bone loss. An increased risk of osteoporosis is seen in populations following this dietary pattern.

I never understood the correlation of dairy/meat consumption and osteoporosis until recently while researching how the body works. The "big" picture wasn't part of my formal academic training in pharmacy school. We were taught to compartmentalize health issues. This was the case with bone health too. We were taught bone loss was caused by a lack of calcium, leading a sedentary lifestyle, and aging. To remedy this loss, we were told to counsel patients to exercise more, supplement with calcium, and ask their doctor about drugs like Fosamax or Reclast. You may have heard of these drugs before. They are known as the bisphosphonates and also include Boniva and Actonel.

Bisphosphonates work by preventing the breakdown of bone in the short term, thereby reducing bone loss. However, this is not necessarily beneficial for bone health in the long term. Our bodies rely on a constant turnover of new bone to replace old, brittle bone in order to prevent fractures. Long-term studies of bisphosphonates have actually shown an increase in atypical leg and hip fractures (stress fractures) because these drugs don't allow for this process to take place as the body was originally designed to do.[23] Hence, they accomplish the exact opposite. They fundamentally weaken large bones found in the leg and hip over time, thereby increasing the risk of stress fractures.

You can better visualize this concept by thinking about repainting the outside of your house. You start by scraping off the old layers of paint before applying a fresh new layer of paint. If this scraping step is skipped, it would lead to the flaking and peeling of the new coat of paint, leaving your house looking like an eye sore after only a few short years. Bones need to be allowed to remodel themselves.

The track record of bisphosphonate therapy speaks for itself when examining these medications success rates. To analyze this, a look at theNNT Reviews is in order (for background information on theNNT please see chapter 3). The physicians at theNNT found that bisphosphonate therapy was of "no benefit" for fracture prevention in post-menopausal women *without* prior history of fractures.[24] Not a single person was helped after three years of therapy in these cases.

In post-menopausal women *with* a history of fractures or very low bone mineral density scores the story is only slightly better.[25] The following is a detailed description of theNNT's findings in such cases after three years of therapy with these medications:

- 94% saw no benefits from taking bisphosphonates
- 5% were helped by avoiding a vertebral fracture (1 in 20)
- 1% were helped by avoiding a hip fracture (1 in 100)
- A small percentage were harmed (stress fractures, osteonecrosis of the jaw, gastrointestinal and musculoskeletal side effects)

Furthermore, theNNT stated at the end of their review that "the studies examined in the Cochrane reviews are industry sponsored. A long history of selective outcome reporting, selective publication, occasionally fraudulent reporting, and dubious methodologic choices all indicate that there is reason to scrutinize and doubt the optimistic claims of these data. Thus these results, while adequate for making clinical decisions, should be considered preliminary unless and until they can be verified on a large scale by parties without a financial stake in the results."

One final health-related issue worth mentioning about dairy consumption is lactose intolerance. It's not uncommon to see others popping Lactaid pills whenever they're about to dip into the ice cream container or down a glass of milk. These individuals have a shortage of the lactase enzyme needed to digest the lactose sugar found in dairy.

Approximately 75 percent of the world's population loses this lactase enzyme after weaning off milk as a child.[26] This loss can lead to a number of painful symptoms including abdominal bloating, cramping, diarrhea, gas, and nausea after drinking a glass of milk. Remove the dairy, substitute a plant-based alternative, and you remove the source of the problem.

Not So Eggscellent

Eggs have become synonymous with breakfast, baking, and the Easter Bunny. Many could not imagine life without them, but if you're looking to improve your health, then these little guys need to stay in the cartons they came in.

Eggs are one of the most concentrated sources of cholesterol in the diet. One large egg has 211 mg of cholesterol in it. This exceeds the 200 mg per day of cholesterol recommended by the Cleveland Clinic for cardiovascular health. Cholesterol is important to human health and is actually required by the body to carry out activities such as building cell membranes, synthesizing hormones, and performing other critical functions. However, the body has the ability to make all the cholesterol it needs without the addition of any added dietary sources of cholesterol.

It's not just the excess cholesterol that's a problem. Eggs are also mostly made up of fat. One large egg contains 63 percent of its calories from fat and, like other animal products, contains a disproportionate amount of pro-inflammatory omega-6 fatty acids compared to anti-inflammatory omega-3 fatty acids. All this adds up to some significant health risks for those who eat eggs.

This was confirmed in the Physician's Health Study out of Harvard. In this study, over 21,000 male physicians were followed for a period of twenty years. Eating just one egg per day resulted in a twofold increased risk of death in those suffering from diabetes.[27] It also increased overall risk of death by 22 percent in those without diabetes.

A review of this same study showed that consuming one or more eggs per day led to a 58 percent increased risk in developing type 2 diabetes.

The news regarding type 2 diabetes and egg consumption is even worse for women. After following over 36,000 women for nearly twelve years the Women's Health Study showed a 77 percent increased risk of developing type 2 diabetes in those who ate one or more eggs per day.[28]

Egg consumption does not bode well for cancer either, specifically prostate cancer. A study in the *American Journal of Clinical Nutrition* in 2010 followed 1,294 men diagnosed with prostate cancer for a period of two years.[29] There was a twofold increased risk of prostate cancer progression in men who ate the most amount of eggs compared to those who ate the least amount. Another study published in 2011 followed over 27,600 cancer-free men for a period of fifteen years. Researchers found that men who consumed an average of just 2.5 eggs per week had an 81 percent increased risk of developing lethal prostate cancer compared to men who consumed only 0.5 eggs per week.[30]

Refined Foods—Stripped of Their Nutrients

Many of the carbohydrates and sugars consumed today in the U.S. have been highly processed and stripped of all their nutrients. These foods are called refined or processed foods. During processing, a majority of the vitamins, minerals, fiber, and phytonutrients are removed.

Food manufacturers will add a small amount of these vitamins and minerals back into the final product to "enrich" them, which leads you to believe they have worthwhile health benefits. They do not. These are nutrient-deficient foods that only succeed in undermining overall health.

In addition to being "enriched," these foods are often loaded down with artificial flavors, colors, and preservatives to make them taste better and last longer on the shelf (yours and the grocer's). By doing this, food manufacturers compromise their own customers' health in exchange for selling more of their product to increase their bottom line. Don't be fooled by these tricks. Short-term satisfaction from consuming nutrient-deficient, highly processed foods will cost you dearly in the long run. Both your health and financial well-being are likely to suffer as you battle a number of chronic diseases resulting from these poor food choices.

America consumes an enormous amount of nutrient-deficient foods. A report from the USDA revealed that, on average, in 2005, Americans consumed 22.7 percent of overall calories from grains, and 89 percent of these calories were from refined grains containing little, if any, nutritional value.[31] This would include items such as white bread, white rice, white pasta, crackers, pastries, cookies, and the like. In addition, added sugars and sweeteners make up another 17.8 percent of total caloric intake—a whopping 30 teaspoons a day or 142 pounds per person per year of added sugars!

There's simply no good reason to consume these kinds of foods in our diet. With over 40 percent of total caloric intake coming from refined foods in the United States, it's easy to see why America has an obesity epidemic and healthcare crisis.

Refined foods and added sugars have been linked to several major diseases including obesity, diabetes, and heart disease. For every 5 percent increase in caloric consumption from refined foods, there's a 33 percent increased risk of having a heart attack.[32] A diet high in processed foods, including sweeteners and refined carbohydrates, has also been shown to increase the incidence of depression.[33] Cutting these nutrient-deficient foods out of your diet and replacing them with a variety of plant-based, whole foods would go a long way in reducing the gluttony of chronic diseases currently experienced in our country.

Limit Sodium Intake

It's widely known that too much sodium in your diet can be harmful, but how much is too much and what do you do after being told by the doctor to go on a low-sodium diet? The first thing most people do is rush home and immediately toss out the salt shaker. Problem solved. Not! Although this is a step in the right direction, it's a far cry from what needs to be done when attempting to reverse the damaging effects of too much sodium in the diet.

The average American consumes 3,466 mg of sodium per day.[34] This is more than double the 1,500 mg/day recommended for most people and well above the upper limit of 2,300 mg/day recommended in the national guidelines. To put this in perspective, one teaspoonful of salt contains 2,300 mg of sodium, so it doesn't take much to exceed the national guidelines.

This excess sodium plays a major role in the development of heart disease and stroke. If the U.S. citizens would reduce their sodium intake by as little as 9.5 percent per year (that's about 350 mg/day per person), it's estimated we would save $32.1 billion in medical costs annually and avert over 513,000 strokes and 480,000 heart attacks each year.[35]

By reducing your sodium intake from the average of 3,500 mg/day to the recommended 1,500 mg/day, you can reduce the risk of having a stroke by 23 percent and the risk of suffering from cardiovascular disease by 17 percent.[36] This is a small price to pay, especially when the alternative could mean financial disaster or permanent disability if you experience one of these horrific events.

As mentioned before, the salt shaker has become our favorite culprit to blame in all of this, but it isn't the major source of sodium in most people's diets when you look at the totality of what we eat. Approximately three-fourths of dietary sodium is actually hidden in the food supply, according to a study in the

> **Approximately three-fourths of dietary sodium is actually hidden in the food supply.**

American Journal of Clinical Nutrition.[37] Data from this study are shown in the chart. The four biggest offenders when it comes to sodium in our diets, besides salt, are processed meats, bread/baked goods, dairy products, and spreads/sauces.

Sources of Dietary Sodium

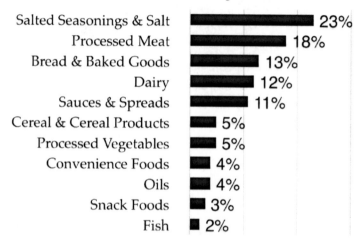

Source	Percent
Salted Seasonings & Salt	23%
Processed Meat	18%
Bread & Baked Goods	13%
Dairy	12%
Sauces & Spreads	11%
Cereal & Cereal Products	5%
Processed Vegetables	5%
Convenience Foods	4%
Oils	4%
Snack Foods	3%
Fish	2%

Reading labels is your best defense in lowering sodium in your diet. Pay attention the next time you pick up a packaged food item from your grocer's shelves and you'll be surprised at what food producers put in there. Avoiding animal-based and processed foods is another easy way to help you achieve the lower recommended intake of 1,500 mg or less per day of sodium. Whole, plant-based foods naturally have only minimal amounts of sodium in them.

While adopting a whole foods, plant-based lifestyle can help prevent heart attacks and stroke, it doesn't provide immunity from all types of stroke. Avoiding animal-based and processed foods will help eliminate the threat of ischemic strokes. These types of strokes happen when a small portion of an atherosclerotic plaque breaks off forming a blood clot. This blood clot eventually gets lodged in a small blood vessel in the brain cutting off subsequent blood supply. A less common type of stroke, called a hemorrhagic stroke, happens when a blood vessel ruptures causing bleeding into the brain. These types of strokes are four times more likely to cause sudden death than ischemic strokes.[38]

Hemorrhagic strokes are also more likely to happen in individuals with "squeaky clean" blood vessels that have little or no atherosclerotic plaque buildup. These plaques, which increase the risk of ischemic stroke, act as a protective barrier against hemorrhagic strokes due to the hardening effect they have on the inside walls of the arteries.[39] Without this protection people with high blood pressure, due to excessive sodium intake, are more prone to their arterial walls rupturing resulting in a hemorrhagic stroke.

Hemorrhagic strokes are two times more prevalent in areas of the world such as Southeast Asia and the Western Pacific than in Europe and North America.[40] Why is that? It's likely due to the high intake of dietary sodium in these parts of the world. Japan, a country known for its traditional diet of mostly plant-based foods (rice, vegetables, and beans), has an extremely high intake of sodium, upwards of 5,300 mg/day for men and 4,500 mg/day for women.[41] Japan's population experiences twice as many hemorrhagic strokes as Americans do.

The important lesson to be learned in all of this is to keep your sodium intake low while adopting a menu of plant-based, whole foods. This will reduce your risk of developing ischemic heart attacks and ischemic strokes. It also gives you the best chance at avoiding hemorrhagic strokes.

The Big Picture of Health and Your Dinner Plate

What you take out of your diet is just as important as what you put into it. Many people love to highlight the positive when it comes to their food choices. *I ate a salad for lunch*, or *We had a side dish of roasted Brussels sprouts for dinner*. But failing to fully grasp the big picture of all your food choices can (and will) disable and kill you prematurely.

The fact of the matter is that bad foods need to be avoided in order to achieve optimal health. While including good (healthy) foods in the diet is always a great thing to do, it's just as important to remove these harmful, disease-causing foods that keep you chronically ill and patronizing our healthcare system. Removing meat, dairy, eggs, and highly refined, processed (junk) foods are a must to accomplish this.

I know you want to do this. Deep down inside you don't want to feel miserable and sick searching hopelessly for answers in the waiting rooms of doctors' offices and long lines at pharmacies. Otherwise, you wouldn't be reading this book in the first place. Making good decisions day in and day out with *all* your food choices will result in the meaningful outcomes you've been looking for when it comes to your health. It's worked for others who've done the same. You can expect it to work for you too if you follow suit.

The Gluten-Free Diet Craze

"After I was diagnosed with celiac disease, I said yes to food, with great enthusiasm... I vowed to taste everything I could eat, rather than focusing on what I could not."

—SHAUNA JAMES AHERN

As the decades have passed so have a multitude of diet crazes. The seventies brought the liquid protein diet, the eighties introduced the low-carb, low-calorie diet, and the nineties led to an explosion of high-protein Atkin's-type diets. Now, with the twenty-first century, we have the gluten-free diet.

You can't walk into a health food store, or even a regular grocery store, today without seeing rows and rows of gluten-free products lining the shelves. There are gluten-free breads, gluten-free crackers, gluten-free pasta, gluten-free cookies, and even gluten-free Johnsonville brats (as if sausages had gluten in them in the first place!). America is sold on the gluten-free craze.

According to a May 2013 article in *Bloomberg Businessweek*, sales of gluten-free products reached $4.2 billion in 2012, and they're projected to keep on climbing to $6.6 billion by 2017.[1] In comparison, sales were a mere $210 million in 2001. That's a huge jump in sales in a relatively short time period.

What's going on here? Are there really that many people developing gluten-related disorders requiring a switch to a gluten-free diet? Or is all of this just hype by the food industry designed to sell more of their overly priced specialty foods to unsuspecting consumers? These questions are at the heart of this chapter. My goal is to explain to you exactly what you need to know in order to determine if going gluten-free is right for you.

Gluten-Related Food Disorders

Gluten is the main structural protein found in wheat, barley, and rye and composed of smaller fragments known as prolamins and glutelin.[2] For most people, gluten proteins can be easily digested without any problems. However, a small portion of the population cannot digest the prolamins found in wheat (gliadin), barley (hordein), and rye (secalin).[3] Unfortunately, this gluten-sensitive group of individuals may develop one of three gluten-related disorders leading to very real, and in some cases, a very serious medical condition.[4] The three gluten-related food disorders are:

- Autoimmune diseases (celiac disease, dermatitis herpetiformis, gluten ataxia)
- Wheat allergy
- Gluten sensitivity

Oats have also been included in the conversation of causing gluten-related disorders. However, this has been shown to be very rare.[5] Oats that have been cross contaminated with wheat during processing are likely the culprits in such cases. Because of this, patients with a gluten-related disorder should avoid oats processed in a factory that also processes wheat, barley, and rye. Otherwise, oats can be part of a healthy gluten-free diet or, at the very least, can be tested in one's diet to see if they cause sensitivities. The three gluten-related disorders are discussed in more detail next.

Autoimmune Diseases
Celiac Disease (CD)
Celiac disease is an autoimmune disorder primarily affecting the small intestine.[6] It is the most common of the autoimmune disorders related to gluten.

In genetically susceptible individuals the intake of dietary gluten causes the body's own immune system to attack the lining of the gut. This leads to inflammation and subsequent damage to the fingerlike projections known as villi found on the surface of the small intestine.[7] Villi play an extremely important role in the digestive process by facilitating the absorption of nutrients into the bloodstream. They also keep toxins and waste products out of the bloodstream. In essence, they are the gatekeepers of everything we eat or drink throughout the day.

The damage inflicted upon the intestinal villi in celiac disease leads to malabsorption problems, which can manifest themselves via a number of classic symptoms—diarrhea, fatty stools, weight loss, abdominal distention, and a state of malnourishment. Other less common symptoms may include growth failure, anemia, osteoporosis, neurological disturbances, dental enamel defects, and persistent nausea and vomiting.[8]

Celiac disease develops over a period of weeks to years of repeated gluten exposure. A diagnosis of celiac disease is achieved by a two-step process. First, blood tests confirm the presence of IgA or IgG antibodies. If antibodies are present, then a biopsy of the small intestine is performed to confirm the diagnosis of celiac disease. It is quite common for the lining of the small intestine to show a flattening out of the villi signifying the damage that's been done during the course of this disease.

Celiac disease is not nearly as common as the food industry wants us to believe. Only 1 percent of the world's population is affected by this disease.[9] In the United States it may be even lower affecting only 0.5 to 1 percent of the population.

Dermatitis Herpetiformis

Dermatitis herpetiformis (DH) is a skin manifestation of celiac disease (sometimes referred to as "skin celiac disease") resulting in a severe, itchy rash followed by the formation of small blisters on the skin.[10] The body literally attacks its own skin in such cases. The blisters formed are often scratched causing them to rupture, dry, and form scabs. The elbows and upper forearms are affected the most (in up to 90 percent of cases). Other sites include the knees, buttocks, neck, scalp, upper back, abdomen, groin, and face.

DH is very rare, occurring only in one of every 10,000 people in both the U.K. and U.S. It is diagnosed by doing a skin biopsy of the papillary dermis—the inner layer of skin found just below the skin's surface. The presence of IgA antibodies provides confirmation of the diagnosis of DH.

Gluten Ataxia

Gluten ataxia (GA) is an autoimmune response to gluten affecting the brain. In GA, the body mistakenly attacks the cerebellum—the part of the brain responsible for balance, motor control, and muscle tone.[11] Sadly, this leads to severe, disabling effects for those suffering from it. These include uncontrolled muscle movements, difficulty walking, loss of fine motor skills, slurred or difficult speech, and rapid, involuntary eye movements.[12]

GA is also a rare disorder. Based on the best available population estimates, it affects approximately 3.4 per 100,000 people.[13]

GA is diagnosed similar to celiac disease by first running blood tests looking for IgA and IgG antibodies. If these are positive, then a biopsy of the small intestine is performed. However, only about a third of patients with GA will show damage to their small intestine on biopsy and less than 10 percent will have gastrointestinal symptoms like those of celiac patients. This makes it difficult for physicians to be 100 percent positive in their diagnosis of the disease. A gluten-free diet is then implemented in hopes of relieving signs and symptoms of GA. If symptoms improve for patients, then GA is the likely diagnosis.

Wheat Allergy

Wheat allergy (WA) is a gluten-related disorder characterized by an allergic reaction to wheat proteins (gliadins). It is not produced by barley proteins (hordein) or rye proteins (secalin), so those who suffer from WA do not need to restrict rye, barley, or oats from their diet.[14]

WA reactions typically occur within minutes to hours of gluten exposure. Patients may experience redness/itchiness of skin; runny nose; hives; wheat-dependent, exercise-induced asthma; occupational asthma (baker's asthma); and in extreme cases anaphylaxis and death. Of these, baker's asthma is the most common form of WA resulting from the inhalation of wheat and cereal flours in bakers. A study of Polish bakery apprentices observed rates of asthma symptoms and runny nose of 8.6 percent and 12.5 percent, respectively, after just two years of being on the job.[15]

The first technique used to diagnose WA is a skin-prick test. However, this method is less than 75 percent accurate due to cross-reactivity with grass pollens, so an oral food challenge is usually implemented to confirm the diagnosis. An oral food challenge involves removing wheat from a person's diet for a period of a few weeks and then reintroducing it to see if WA symptoms reoccur. Another method used to confirm the diagnosis of WA is to perform a blood test to detect IgE antibodies. The detection of IgE antibodies warrants a 74 percent positive predictive value for the diagnosis of WA.[16]

Worldwide prevalence of WA is extremely low. Rates as low as 0.21 percent have been reported in Japanese adults, while rates of 0.2–0.9 percent have been noted in adult populations of Europe and the United States.[17]

Gluten Sensitivity

Nonceliac gluten sensitivity, or gluten sensitivity (GS) for short, is a condition similar to celiac disease, but with no known autoimmune component to it.[18] There is also no evidence of an allergy component to GS, like WA has.[19]

GS usually occurs within hours to days of ingesting gluten-containing foods. Patients can experience an array of symptoms including abdominal pain, eczema and/or rash, headache, "foggy mind," fatigue, diarrhea, depression, anemia, numbness of the extremities, and joint pain.

As mentioned, there is no autoimmune component to GS. This means the body does not attack itself as it does in cases of celiac disease or DH. No antibodies show up on blood tests, and the lining of the gut appears completely normal upon biopsy. GS is literally a medical condition finding itself in "no man's land" with no official diagnostic criteria to confirm its presence.

So doctors and patients are left with a trial-and-error approach in diagnosing and treating the condition. This is done by implementing a gluten-free diet in hopes of eliminating the symptoms encountered by it. If symptoms disappear, then GS is diagnosed. If not, then GS is ruled out.

GS is thought to be six times more prevalent than celiac disease, making it the most prevalent of all gluten-related disorders.[20]

When to Go Gluten-Free

Where does this leave us? Should you wake up tomorrow, wipe out your pantry, and start all over with nothing but gluten-free products? Or should you include gluten-containing foods as part of a healthy diet?

If you have a gluten-related medical condition as described in this chapter, then it is important, if not critical, to adopt a gluten-free diet as part of an overall whole foods, plant-based lifestyle to greatly increase your chances of living a healthy, disease-free life.

Gluten-related disorders are real. They lead to unnecessary pain and suffering and can be fatal in rare cases. However, their prevalence is blown way out of proportion when looking at the population as a whole. Even our best estimates translate into at most 10–11 percent of the world's population affected by one of these disorders, and this is being generous. In addition, the most serious of all the gluten-related disorders—celiac disease—affects only 1 percent of the world's population. These numbers are a far cry from the 29 percent of Americans trying to avoid gluten because they "think" it's the right thing to do for their health.[21]

The reality of the situation is that gluten-containing foods—wheat, barley, and rye—are safe for at least 90 percent or more of the population. They should serve as a healthy addition to the majority of people's diets based on the best available evidence. Gluten-containing foods are an inexpensive source of essential calories, fiber, and a number of vitamins, minerals, and other phytonutrients important in maintaining optimal health.

Gluten-containing foods have also been shown to positively influence the bacterial colonization of the gut as well.[22] This results in more "good" bacteria and less "bad" bacteria colonizing the colon supporting a healthier immune system in the long run. It would be unfortunate and unwise for an entire population to forgo the benefits of gluten-containing foods simply because of a scientifically unfounded diet craze.

Keep the Big Picture in Mind

For those who have a confirmed medical condition requiring the avoidance of gluten, the chart on the next page can help you delineate between gluten-containing vs. gluten-free grains. A number of whole grain products serve as viable substitutes to wheat, barley, and rye. Including these grains as part of a whole foods, plant-based lifestyle will help you attain optimal health while providing both satisfaction and satiety to your daily menu.

Let's view the gluten-free topic in context with the bigger picture. Many people are fooled into believing going gluten-free will magically take care of their health issues. Unfortunately, this is not the case. What often happens is these same individuals end up filling their grocery carts full of gluten-free processed junk foods (along with animal-based and other processed foods) thinking they are doing right by their diet only to find out they're not. Ultimately, ill health and chronic disease rage on as America gets caught up in "healthy" living by going gluten-free.

In the next chapter, I will explain how to avoid deceptive marketing tactics of the corporate food giants, which suck you in to buying these junk foods. You'll learn how to steer clear of all packaged processed foods—gluten-free or not—as you continue to expand your knowledge of what a whole foods, plant-based lifestyle looks like in practical terms.

Gluten-Containing Grains	Gluten-Free Grains and Flours
Wheat Wheat varieties (bulgur, couscous, dinkel, durum, einkorn, emmer, farro, farina, freekeh, fu, gliadin, glutenin, graham flour, kamut, matzo, seitan, semolina, spelt, wheat berry, wheat germ, and cracked wheat) Barley Rye	Amaranth Arrowroot Buckwheat (cousin of rhubarb) Corn (maize) Dasheen flour Job's tears Kasha (buckwheat groats) Kudzu Millet Oats* Potato flour Quinoa Rice (all varieties) Sago Sorghum Soy flour Tapioca flour Taro flour Teff Wild Rice

*Oats are gluten-free but are often contaminated with wheat during growing or processing.

Putting a Healthy Lifestyle into Practice

"When it comes to eating right and exercising, there is no 'I'll start tomorrow.' Tomorrow is disease."

—TERRI GUILLEMETS

K nowing what's right for yourself and doing what's right for yourself are two different things. You now know how to live a long, happy, and disease-free life. The only task remaining is your willingness to put this knowledge into action. This chapter is written with this in mind. I want to make things easier for you by giving you practical tips in achieving your health-related goals.

The first and foremost action you need to do is implement the *Food For Health* eating guide from chapter 9. This should serve as the centerpiece for your daily meals and snacks. Study it, memorize it, and get to know it as if it were woven into your very DNA because this guide is the most crucial part of your future success. Without understanding this concept, the physical and biological processes of the human body will leave you searching for answers as your food selections once again sabotage any well-meaning intentions you may have had.

Give It a Month

Everyone is different and achieves success using various methods. What works for one person may or may not work for another. Some people transition slowly into a plant-based lifestyle. They find it's too overwhelming to go cold turkey. Others have no problem diving right in and never looking back as they say goodbye to animal-based and processed foods forever. There's no right or wrong way to transition. I'm not going to tell you which approach is best for you because only you can determine this. The more profound changes you make, the more profound results you'll see in your health.

If you currently suffer from a chronic disease, then your best bet is to go all in. You can't afford to experience a fatal heart attack, a crippling stroke, or similar catastrophic event. These ordeals have permanent consequences and can occur at any time. By switching immediately to a whole foods, plant-based lifestyle you'll start to see immediate results as your body begins to repair the damage caused by years of eating a Western diet. Within a matter of days or a few short weeks, your blood pressure will normalize, your cholesterol levels will come down, the weight will come off, and you'll start having more energy.

> The more profound changes you make, the more profound results you'll see.

One easy way to start is to give this new lifestyle a try for one full month. A commitment of just thirty days is a mere blip on the map when compared to the time spent getting to this stage of your life. You've more than likely spent thirty days or more on various programs and diets that didn't work anyway, so you really have nothing to lose by making this new lifestyle change for such a short period of time. As you start to feel and see the results firsthand, the excitement will build, and this will act as motivation to keep you going. Soon, your newly formed habits will turn into just another day of healthy eating, filled with delicious new plant-based recipes. You'll be wondering why you didn't switch sooner.

Plan Ahead

Like anything new in life it takes time to learn new processes. Once you accomplish any transition, you never think twice about the time spent performing your new activities. It becomes routine and the same holds true for your eating habits. Switching to a whole foods, plant-based lifestyle will become a normal way of eating for you after only three to four weeks.

The best way to make this transition successful is to plan ahead. Taking just fifteen minutes a week to plan out a weekly menu will result in a lot less stress. If you're like many people and tend to eat the same things for breakfast and lunch every day, then half your work is already done. This leaves only dinner to worry about. Most people tend to rotate between their favorite ten to fifteen meals regardless of what type of food they normally eat, so planning ahead really isn't as much of a monumental task as it sounds.

To start planning ahead, take out a piece of paper and write down the days of the week. Pick two to four recipes that appeal to you. Pencil them in for dinner throughout the week. When preparing and cooking these meals, make a little extra to have leftovers available for the remaining days of the week. Leftovers are quick, easy, and quite delicious, plus they make life much less stressful because you won't have to worry about cooking every day. Continue filling out the remainder of your meal plan until all gaps are filled. Here's a sample meal plan to help you get started.

One Day Sample Meal Plan
Breakfast   • Oatmeal with cinnamon, walnuts, raisins, and blueberries   • Watermelon slices   • Whole grain toast with almond butter
Mid-Morning Snack   • Apple
Lunch   • Spinach and Arugula salad with a variety of freshly chopped veggies   • Hummus, lettuce, and tomato wrap   • Plum
Mid-Afternoon Snack   • Chocolate coconut oat bars
Dinner   • Black bean burritos   • Spanish rice with roasted tomatoes   • Peach cobbler

You can do many other things to make the transition to healthier eating simpler and more enjoyable. Here are a few tips to help you out:

- Dedicate a few hours a week to preparing and chopping fruits and veggies for storage in ready-made containers to be used throughout the week.
- Keep an ongoing grocery list as you make your way through the week.
- Try out various slow cooker recipes and let the cooker do the work for you as you spend your days tending to other activities.
- Make dinner a family event so you can spend more quality time together as you prepare, cook, and eat healthy meals with one another.
- Buy prepared foods—canned beans, frozen fruits/veggies, presliced/chopped fresh produce with no added salt or sugar.
- Prepare your workday lunch the night before so you can "grab and go" as you run out the door the next morning.
- Use a food processor to save time slicing, dicing, blending, pureeing, and shredding your favorite foods.
- Don't spend so much time measuring exact amounts of spices and herbs to add to recipes; instead add selected ingredients to taste.

Another piece of advice to keep life more manageable is to enjoy simple, easy meals when you don't feel like cooking. Throwing a sweet potato in the oven or making instant brown rice and serving these items with a side of steamed veggies and heated beans makes a delicious meal with little effort. Not everything has to be a gourmet meal to be healthy.

Grocery Shopping and Label Reading

The path to excellent health begins with a powerful new grocery list, but this is only as good as the person using it. Grocery aisles can be deceptive so it's essential to know how to navigate them. The first step in mastering the art of shopping is to target the produce section. Foods in this section usually don't have barcodes on them, just as nature intended them.

Choose organic, locally grown, fresh fruits and vegetables from nearby farms or neighborhood farmers' markets if possible. These are of the highest quality and offer the greatest benefits. They typically cost the same or even less than matching items found in local grocery stores. If this isn't possible or seasonal, then fresh and frozen vegetables from your local supermarket is the next best thing.

Frozen fruits and vegetables actually lock in their nutrients shortly after being picked or harvested, which often makes them better choices than fresh produce, especially if produce is shipped in from thousands of miles away to your local grocer's shelves. Canned fruits and vegetables are a viable third option behind fresh and frozen products. They should be low in sodium or have no added salt or sugar. Remember, the quicker fruits and vegetables make their way from the farm to your plate, the better. They'll taste more flavorful and provide more nutritional value as well.

The safest area to shop from as you make your way through the supermarket is the perimeter of the store. That's where you'll find the most healthful foods. However, if you venture into the middle of the store aisles, then it's important to know how to effectively decipher the Nutrition Facts label.

The graphic below highlights four specific lines. These are the only lines you need to pay attention to on a label. Don't worry about the remaining numbers and percentages. They'll only manage to confuse you. In addition, you'll need to read the ingredients list. Follow these tips to ensure the purchasing of healthful items. Familiarize yourself with these tips (see next page) and commit them to memory. They can literally save your life.

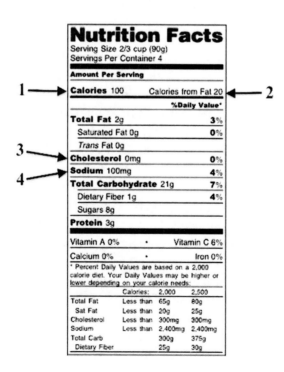

Label Reading

1. **Fat Content.** Buy items with no more than 20 percent of their calories from fat. To calculate, compare the calories (Item 1) to the calories from fat (Item 2) and make sure this doesn't exceed 20 percent. The label provided contains 100 calories per serving. Therefore, 20 calories or less should come from fat, which is exactly the case in this example. If a product were to contain 150 calories per serving, then no more than 30 calories should come from fat. There are a few items to make an exception for including nuts and seeds, their respective products (almond butter, peanut butter, and other nut butters), and plant-based milks (soy milk and almond milk, for example). These items, when consumed in small quantities, can be a healthy addition to a whole foods, plant-based menu.

2. **Cholesterol Content.** There is no measurable amount of cholesterol in plant-based foods. In contrast, all animal-based foods contain cholesterol. When looking at cholesterol content on a label (Item 3) make sure it always says 0 mg. If it says anything other than zero, then the item in question contains animal products and is better left on the shelf.

3. **Sodium Content.** As pointed out in chapter 10, the recommended amount of sodium per day is 1,500 mg or less for most adults, with an upper limit of 2,300 mg per day. Most people exceed this upper limit. Most individuals also consume approximately 2,000 calories per day, give or take a few. With this being the case, the easiest way to control your sodium intake is to compare the calories (Item 1) to the sodium content (Item 4). Make sure the amount of sodium per serving is equal to or less than the number of calories per serving. In this case, the product contains 100 calories per serving and 100 mg of sodium per serving so it passes the test. By following this tip, if you consume the average of 2,000 calories per day, then you'll never go over the upper limit of 2,300 mg of sodium per day, and it's more likely you'll be at or under the recommended limit of 1,500 mg per day.

4. **Read the Ingredient List**. It's also imperative to read the ingredient list when looking at a nutrition label. A majority of products have a list of ingredients a mile long, most of which many people have never heard of. This is a good sign these products have been heavily processed. It's best to avoid such products. In addition, avoid products with harmful fats and added sugars, or at the very least, make sure these ingredients are not listed in the first five items on the ingredient list:

- **Harmful Fats.** Saturated animal fats (lard, butter, chicken fat), oils (partially hydrogenated oils, palm oil, coconut oil, palm kernel oil, cottonseed oil), and man-made saturated fats (margarine and shortening)
- **Added Sugars.** High fructose corn syrup, evaporated cane juice, dehydrated honey, sugar, honey, brown rice syrup, corn syrup, molasses, cane sugar, maltodextrose, and others

One final important topic pertains to selecting whole grain products. When buying these products, make sure you look for the words *whole, cracked, stone-ground, rolled,* or *graham flour.* If the product contains 100 percent whole grain ingredients, then these words are legally required to be present. *Whole wheat* bread is a legitimate whole grain product, but *wheat* bread is not. This is refined food made from white flour.

Finding Substitutes

Meat Substitutes

Meat is simple to find alternatives to. Beans, along with other legumes, are an excellent way to replace meat in your diet. They come with a healthy dose of fiber to help fill you up. Whether preparing chili, tacos, burritos, soups, stews, or other dishes, it's easy to substitute beans for meat in a recipe. Tempeh or tofu can also be used as an alternative to meat. They tend to take on the flavor of whatever they're seasoned with. Marinate or glaze them with your favorite sauce and enjoy them as a grilled side addition, in stir-fries, or crumbled up in various casseroles.

Finally, another great meat replacement is seitan. Seitan is often referred to as "wheat meat" since it is made from gluten. If you don't have a gluten disorder, then this can make a suitable alternative to meat. It can be used to make burgers, added to Asian-style noodle dishes, or as a part of grilled kabobs.

Dairy Substitutes

Numerous varieties of plant-based milks now line the shelves of most grocery stores. Soy, hemp, rice, oat, and almond milks are all worth trying. Coconut milk is available as well, but it's very high in fat so I don't recommend this product as part of a health-promoting diet. Many plant-based milks are sweetened, so it's best to use them as a condiment to your meals rather than drinking them by the glassful. You can skip the added sugars too and buy the unsweetened versions if desired.

Imitation "cheese" products are now everywhere, but it's important to read labels when selecting these items. Some contain casein, the main protein found in cow's milk. As mentioned in chapter 10, casein is a known cancer promoter. Make sure this is not found in the ingredient list.

Many of the soy "cheeses" and other commercial cheese alternatives contain high amounts of sodium. Use them sparingly, if at all. The safest replacement for cheese is to make your own using tofu or nutritional yeast as a base. Plenty of recipes can be found online. I even include one with my Veggie Pita Pizza recipe in this book. Nutritional yeast is a great replacement for Parmesan cheese and can be found in most local health food stores. It has the appearance of a flaky powder, which makes it easy to sprinkle on pasta dishes or other recipes.

Egg Replacements

Eggs are one of the easiest items to find substitutes for. It's important to understand what an egg is being used for in a recipe to find the best-suited replacement. Recipes calling for more than three eggs are more of a challenge when trying to find a replacement, but it can be done. If a recipe calls for just one egg, many times it can be omitted or a small amount of water can be added instead. The chart below provides suitable substitutes for egg replacements.

Egg's Purpose	Replace 1 Egg with One of the Following
Main ingredient (omelette, quiche, frittata)	¼ cup blended silken tofu
Binding agent (cookies, muffins, pancakes, biscuits)	½ mashed banana ¼ cup applesauce ¼ cup soy yogurt ¼ cup mashed potatoes ¼ cup pureed pears ⅓ cup pumpkin puree 1 tbsp ground flaxseed + 3 tbsp water
Leavening agent (cakes)	1 tbsp vinegar + 1 tsp baking soda 1 tsp baking powder
Thickening agent (custards, pie filling)	¼ cup blended silken tofu

Oil and Butter Substitutes

By now you're well aware of the fact that all oils should be avoided if you wish to achieve optimal health. This can be challenging for many people as oil is used for multiple purposes such as sautéing vegetables or as part of various recipes. To solve the problem of sautéing with oil, just replace it with the same amount of water, low-sodium vegetable stock, or cooking wine. Use nonstick cookware to cut down on the need for a sautéing additive.

In recipes use the following tips. If a tablespoonful or less of oil is called for, just omit it. Most of the time you'll never know the difference. If a substitute is needed, then try applesauce, prune puree, or ground flaxseed meal. Six tablespoons of prune puree replaces half cup of oil; three parts of flaxseed meal can be substituted for one part oil; applesauce can be replaced in equal amounts. These same tricks can be used to replace butter in recipes.

Eating Out and Dining In

Since food is often the focal point of our social lives, it's not uncommon to attend a dinner gathering or go out to eat with family members and friends, which can pose certain challenges for those living a plant-based lifestyle, but these challenges can easily be met.

Attending a Gathering

When asked to attend a lunch or dinner gathering at someone's house, be upfront and open with them. Share with the host your new way of eating and explain why this is important to you. Most people will be supportive if you're genuine and sincere with your intentions.

To ease their anxieties, offer to bring a healthy appetizer, your favorite plant-based dish, or a fruit and veggie platter for everyone to enjoy. By doing so, you'll have something to eat and may just surprise others by how delicious plant-based dishes can be. Avoid bringing up your new lifestyle at the table unless specifically asked by others. Instead, focus on their stories and passions in life. It's amazing how well others warm up to you and quickly forget about your new way of eating when you do this.

Another tip is to eat a snack before attending gatherings. Arriving with something in your stomach will make you less likely to give in to the temptations of eating unhealthy foods. If worse comes to worse, you can always raid the refrigerator once you return home. Before leaving and throughout the dinner party always remain thankful to your host for everything. Remember, the most important aspect of a social gathering is connecting with others and sharing experiences about life, love, and happiness. Nobody will remember what you ate or didn't eat at a particular event, but I guarantee you they'll remember how you made them feel.

Dining Out

Keeping it healthy while eating out can be made easy with a little planning and familiarity with the local landscape. A wonderful website known as www.HappyCow.net makes finding healthy, friendly eating establishments practically effortless. Their database spans the entire globe containing thousands of plant-based friendly cafes and restaurants at the simple click of a button. It's a helpful resource to use, especially when traveling to unfamiliar places. You can also find some hidden treasures in your own backyard. They may just become your new favorite hangout.

Our world is becoming much more friendly when it comes to offering plant-based meals to customers. The increased interest in this lifestyle has led to some well-known restaurants providing healthier options. Some of these national establishments include Sweet Tomatoes, Crispers, Chipotle, and Moe's, just to name a few. Most other popular chains will offer at least one plant-based-friendly meal option on their menu.

Don't be afraid to ask for what you want. Many times the chef can come up with something to impress your taste buds while keeping it healthy at the same time. Make sure to always ask if they can prepare your food without salt or oil too. When ordering pasta or bread, request whole wheat items if available. The more customers make these kinds of requests, the more available healthy foods will become for everyone.

Another option when dining out is to think globally. Many regions of the world have lived on plant-based foods for centuries, and the absence of chronic, degenerative diseases experienced by their people speaks volumes to the health-promoting aspects of their diet. When trying different ethnic cuisines, ask the staff if there are any dairy products in their items and avoid those dishes or see if they can make them without dairy. It may be as easy as leaving the cheese off a salad, appetizer, or entree. Once again, see if their food can be prepared without any added salt or oils.

Enjoy choosing from a wide range of ethnic foods including the following cuisines—Mexican, Chinese, Japanese, Vietnamese, Ethiopian, Indian, Latin American, Mediterranean, and even Thai. Whether it's bean burritos, sushi and miso soup, or vegetable pad Thai, there's bound to be something that appeals to your unique tastes. You won't be sacrificing any enjoyment. You'll just be adding health to your new way of eating when dining out.

A Nation of Addicts

"You know you are addicted to a food if despite knowing it is bad for you and despite wanting to change, you still keep eating it. Addiction means that a craving has more control over your behavior than you do."

—KATHY FRESTON

More people die from the result of an addiction each year in America than from any other cause. I'm not talking about the one out of every five deaths due to tobacco and nicotine abuse each year in the United States.[1] Nor am I speaking of the tens of thousands of individuals who die each year due to their dependence on drugs and alcohol.

The addiction I'm referring to affects far more people than smoking, drugs, and alcohol. This addiction goes seemingly unnoticed by those who suffer from it and tends to fly under the radar among the news media in our country. It also evades the medical community that attempts to treat it. Furthermore, the debilitating and often fatal events resulting from this addiction are actually fueled by our government officials who pass laws to encourage the continuation of it.

I'm talking about America's addiction to the foods we eat. More than half of the leading causes of death in the United States are either entirely or in part due to the rich foods of the Standard American Diet.

We are a nation of addicts who've been taken hostage by our internal brain chemistry as we seek ways to get our next hit off three main ingredients—fat, sugar, and salt. These substances hijack the pleasure centers in our brain in much the same way that cocaine, amphetamines, and other drugs hijack the brains of drug addicts.[2] Unfortunately, many people end up engaging in these behaviors multiple times a day, seven days a week, 365 days a year, which brings us to the very definition of addiction: "persistent compulsive use of a substance known by the user to be harmful."[3]

Our addiction to unhealthy foods is not due to a lack of willpower. It is a disease with a biological explanation just like any other addiction. It requires acceptance by those facing it, along with a desire to move forward to overcome it. This chapter will explain why we desire foods rich in salt, sugar, and fat as well as explain what's happening inside the brain to cause this dependency. By gaining an understanding of what's occurring on the inside of the body, it will better allow for those affected by this addiction to take the steps needed to break the cycle of unhealthy habits.

Nature's Perfect Feedback Loop

Human beings, along with other species in the animal kingdom, were designed to engage in rewarding behaviors. The positive feedback loop embedded within us was not a mistake by Mother Nature. In fact, this reward system is absolutely necessary for our survival.

Doug Lisle, PhD, and Alan Goldhamer, DC, allude to this in their book *The Pleasure Trap*.[4] In it, they've coined the term *motivational triad*, which is nature's way of ensuring the survival and reproduction of any given species. This motivational triad consists of three components—seeking pleasure, avoiding pain, and conserving energy.

It makes perfect sense that if we engage in activities that accomplish these three things, then we'll experience both health and happiness and the success that comes with them. We'll also be able to carry forward our family genes by reproducing offspring who can then continue this same process. We were meant to enjoy the acts of eating, sleeping, and having sex for these very reasons.

In recent times, however, we've learned to shortcut this natural feedback loop in order to experience feelings of intense pleasure and reward. Drugs, alcohol, gambling, smoking, casual sex, compulsive shopping, and eating rich Western foods are all prime examples. They result in enormous pleasure in the short term while compromising our long-term ability to be happy, healthy, and successful. A heroin addict will go to any lengths to experience the rush from taking a single hit, even if it means getting thrown in prison or, worse yet, ending up dead. The euphoric high is always more important than life itself from the drug addict's perspective.

The same holds true for other detrimental behaviors. For example, eating the Standard American Diet of French fries, ice cream, and fried chicken can provide enormous gratification in the short term but comes with its own set of long-term health consequences. For this reason, it's important to understand the difference between activities that offer both short-term pleasure and long-term health versus activities that result in short-term satisfaction at the expense of our long-term health. The rich, Western diet accomplishes the latter. It has the same harmful effects as addiction to heroin. It just takes longer for the ill health effects to occur in most cases. This is the reason why cardiovascular disease, cancer, and diabetes are so prevalent among our population today.

Rich Western foods provide an immediate high just like heroin but only on a smaller scale with less intensity. These foods cause our body to form recurrent cravings much like illicit street drugs do. This ultimately turns into an addiction after repeated exposure. It's why many people cannot fathom the thought of giving up cheese or ice cream for the rest of their lives. It's also why people make a midnight run to the nearest Kwik-E-Mart to get a Twinkie fix. Nobody ever makes a midnight dash for a fresh head of broccoli and hummus dip.

Both of these snacks can be delicious in their own right. However, the cravings leading us to seek Twinkies in the wee hours of the morning go far beyond mental toughness and straight to a handful of powerful neurotransmitters working overtime in your brain. Let me explain how that works.

A Brain under Siege

Dopamine is a neurotransmitter that plays a critical role inside the brain. It is involved in many important functions including voluntary movement, cognition, learning, memory, and reward-seeking behavior.[5] These different processes occur in various parts of the brain. The role of dopamine most pertinent to the topic of food addiction is the reward-seeking function. The reward center of the brain is centered in the nucleus accumbens, found in the middle of the brain. The prefrontal cortex, located in the front of the brain, also plays a role in this process but to a lesser extent.

When a drug addict takes his first snort of cocaine, this causes immense pleasure. This intense high results from a surge of dopamine released into the nucleus accumbens.[6] This surge of dopamine is effectively acting as a form of currency for the brain's reward center much like money acts as a form of currency in a person's bank account. If you were to win the lottery, you would experience intense feelings of excitement and pleasure as a mountain of cash is deposited into your bank account. This feeling would wear off eventually as the money becomes depleted from spending it.

The cocaine addict experiences this same loss of excitement as the drug gets flushed out of his system. He then becomes desperate to find his next hit to experience the next high. Over time, with repeated exposure, an addiction forms and tolerance levels rise requiring more of the drug to get the same effect. This snowball effect is how a one-time encounter with a powerful street drug turns into a daily nightmare of cravings and addictions with serious consequences for the end user.

The same exact scenario plays out for hundreds of millions of Americans as a diet high in fat and sugar causes a dopamine onslaught to their brain's reward center.[7,8] This happens multiple times per day each time we eat. Salted foods are also thought to stimulate opiate and dopamine receptors in the brain causing addictive-like behaviors.[9] These highly palatable foods act to override the body's natural feedback loop responsible for determining the amount of calories needed to meet our daily energy requirements.[10] Therefore, we no longer experience a feeling of fullness that's accompanied with having enough to eat, which results in overeating increasing the risk of becoming overweight. As you already know, excess weight is a big risk factor in the development of many chronic diseases.

A handful of appetite-stimulating compounds have been found to play an important role in the process of increasing dopamine levels in the brain.[11] They're known as orexigenic peptides and include galanin, enkephalin, dynorphin, and orexin. These compounds act as messengers between brain cells relaying what actions need to be taken depending on how they are activated.

The problem occurs when these peptides are activated by circulating fats (triglycerides) in the blood from eating a high-fat diet. This process overrides the body's positive feedback loop responsible for telling our brain when we're "full." As a result, we continue to seek out and consume more dietary fat. Thousands of years ago when food was scarce, this may have been important to one's survival, but in today's world of unlimited food supply it has deadly consequences.

These same neuropeptides also play a role in alcohol consumption. Galanin, enkephalin, and dynorphin are all increased by ethanol ingestion.[12] There is a corresponding increase in triglyceride and blood alcohol levels due to this effect further promoting the consumption of additional alcoholic beverages and high-fat foods.[13] This can quickly become a problem because alcohol is a high-calorie beverage containing nearly double the amount of calories per gram than that of carbohydrates and proteins. When you couple this with the fact it also increases the brain's desire to eat foods high in fat, it's no wonder a person is able to consume way more calories than they should in the first place.

Sugar is another major culprit when it comes to food cravings and addictions. As mentioned before, sugar consumption leads to sharp increases in dopamine levels in the brain. It also binds to and activates opioid receptors leading to cravings and addictions similar to those of cocaine and morphine, only on a much smaller scale.[14] This leads to bingeing on foods and beverages high in sugar and causes one to experience opiate-like withdrawal symptoms when attempting to get off these foods.[15] This is part of the reason why someone trying to break his or her soda habit is so irritable and anxious. The added withdrawal symptoms from caffeine make this task even more daunting.

Hooked on Dairy

Along with having the addictive properties of being high-fat foods, dairy products also contain a certain substance that provides that little extra something to get people hooked on them. This extra something is an opioidlike substance called beta-casomorphin. It's derived from the breakdown of casein, the main protein in cow's milk. Beta-casomorphin produces a small morphinelike effect by activating opioid receptors in the brain.[16]

This concept actually has some biological relevance to it but not as it pertains to humans drinking cow's milk. It turns out human breast milk also contains beta-casomorphins. These substances act to attract newborns to their mother's milk, especially in the first year of life, which was intended to foster healthy growth and development through proper nutrition for the infant. A mother's milk was designed to be nature's perfect food when used for her own species.

However, when we drink another species' milk, this no longer holds true—a theory that was revealed in a study comparing the effect of human breast milk versus cow's milk formula on infants.[17] Researchers found that both groups of infants had elevated levels of beta-casomorphins after being fed either breast milk or a formula derived from cow's milk, but the cow's milk group experienced problems in the normal maturation process. This group showed a delay in psychomotor development (relationship between cognitive function and physical movement), which can increase the risk of diseases such as autism.[17,18] The breast-fed infants showed no such developmental issues or health consequences as a result of their nutritional intake.

Dairy is not an easy thing to give up and for good reason. Milk and cheese are high in fat, contain morphinelike substances, and in some cases have extra salt and sugar added to their final products. Cheese in particular contains approximately 70 percent of its calories from fat. This is a big reason why it's one of the hardest foods to say goodbye to. It was actually the last animal-based food I gave up in my quest to adopt a plant-based lifestyle.

Breaking the Cycle of Addiction

Feeling great and living a disease-free life are at the top of everyone's list if you ask them. Nobody ever wants to experience pain and suffering. There's not a smoker on the face of the planet who wants to get lung cancer. Nor is there an alcoholic who wishes to suffer from liver disease or a drug addict who wants to end up dead of an overdose. Human beings innately appreciate a state of feeling good and living well, but this doesn't keep them from engaging in habits that undermine their health.

Coming to a realization that certain behaviors are detrimental to your health is the first step in breaking the cycle of unhealthy habits. Sadly, many people are not even aware of the addictive properties of the foods they consume every day. Reading this chapter is a smart first step in overcoming this barrier. The more you understand about a topic, the better prepared you are to face the problem when it arises. Once you realize there's a problem, then it's time to move forward in a positive direction.

Understand that moving forward may also mean experiencing some rough patches along the way, especially in the beginning. Because highly palatable foods have the same addictive properties as drugs and alcohol, they can also produce undesirable side effects when withdrawing from them. Stress, anxiety, and depressed moods are all common withdrawal symptoms when giving up these foods in your diet.[19] This is normal. It is also temporary.

The degree to which these symptoms occur usually correlates to how much rich Western food a person currently consumes. Fortunately, these symptoms only take about three to four weeks to disappear once a person switches to a healthier way of eating. The best way to do this is to follow my *Food For Health* eating guide.

Removing highly palatable foods from an unhealthy diet has also been shown to change your taste preferences over time. Just as an individual needs more drugs to satisfy her needs, an individual who regularly consumes high amounts of salt, sugar, and fat will need higher amounts of these substances to satisfy her taste buds.[20,21] Once you switch to healthier plant-based foods, your taste buds "open up" as they become more sensitive to these ingredients. As a matter of fact, you'll actually be completely resetting your taste preferences when switching to a plant-based lifestyle.

A study analyzing a reduction in sodium intake in adults shows how this concept works.[22] After five months on a low-sodium diet, subjects perceived a marked increase in intensity levels to salt. A significant reduction in the preferred level of sodium was shown in participants throughout the course of the study. In other words, the more study participants avoided salt/sodium in their diet, the less they needed it to satisfy their taste preferences.

Understanding what happens while transitioning from addictive foods to healthy foods is the first step to overcoming these cravings. The next critical objective is to make these changes habit forming. I mentioned it can take three to four weeks to get over the withdrawal period from eliminating addictive foods. It takes the same amount of time to turn new behaviors into sustainable habits. The knowledge provided in this chapter and the tips provided in chapter 12 were designed to do just that for you.

Overcoming the physical dependence that animal-based and processed foods have on your mind and body is now within your grasp. It no longer has to be the frightening experience that you once feared.

But So-and-So Said—
Debunking Common Beliefs

"It's bizarre that the produce manager is more important to my children's health than the pediatrician."
—MERYL STREEP

witching to a whole foods, plant-based lifestyle can be life altering. Its foundation is backed by scientific evidence, and its success is paralleled by the ensuing clinical results seen by the patients and doctors who practice it on a daily basis. Although the general public and many healthcare professionals are opening up to this approach, it has yet to be put into practice on a mass scale. Some of this reluctance may be fueled by the many myths that exist between the world of plant-based nutrition and what people perceive it to be.

It's perfectly normal to have questions and become skeptical when faced with new information. Many times the conclusions we come to are founded on popular beliefs instead of cold hard facts. Confusion develops leading to misguided interpretation of what is true and what is not true. This only serves to turn people off before they even get started on their new journey. Unfortunately, this robs them of a secure, healthy future. My goal is to address these concerns by presenting the scientific facts behind the most popular myths about plant-based nutrition.

Where Do You Get Your Protein?

By far, this is one of the most commonly asked questions from others when they learn about living a plant-based lifestyle. Everyone is worried about not getting enough protein, especially if they leave meat and dairy out of their diet. The concern over getting enough protein is indeed a legitimate one. Protein is absolutely essential for humans to stay alive and function properly. There are hundreds of thousands of different kinds of proteins in the human body, and they all play an important role. Proteins function as enzymes and cellular signaling molecules in the body, as well as key structural components in our muscle and connective tissues.[1]

The importance of getting enough protein has been overemphasized as far back as when it was discovered in 1838 by Gerardus Mulder.[2] Then and now, protein has been regarded as the most revered of all nutrients and considered more important than carbohydrates, fats, and vitamins and minerals. The problem is not that we don't get enough protein, but that we get too much, especially from animal sources, which leads to a decline in overall health.

Epidemiological studies have shown a diet rich in meat protein increases the risk of kidney stone formation.[3] There's also a higher incidence in cardiovascular-related events in those who have higher protein intakes in their diet.[4] Animal-based proteins have been shown to increase the rates of various cancers as covered in chapter 5.

In 2002, the World Health Organization (WHO) released a publication titled *Protein and Amino Acid Requirements in Human Nutrition.*[5] In this publication they discussed the daily protein requirements for adults after analyzing the evidence-based scientific literature. They found even after allowing for a "safety zone" above the minimum energy requirements needed by adults that an intake of 0.66 grams/kg/day of protein was more than sufficient to meet the body's needs. This equals approximately 5 percent of total calories coming from protein.

For individuals with an ideal body weight of 120 to 175 pounds, this is equivalent to 36 to 53 grams of protein per day. Yet the typical American adult consumes between 66 and 91 grams of protein per day, nearly double what is actually needed.[6] Those following a plant-based lifestyle intake more than adequate amounts of protein at 60 to 80 grams per day.[7] Not getting enough is not the problem. If anything, we're getting too much protein.

Protein requirements for athletes have been a concern for many individuals who train or participate in competitive sports. Again, the popular consensus of "more is better" does not always hold up when it comes to protein intake. It is true athletes require more protein than the average person to recover from their respective sport or activity. The belief they need to consume massive amounts of egg whites, meat, and protein shakes to meet these needs is not true.

A study assessing the actual protein replacement needs for strength training athletes found a daily intake of 1.41 grams/kg/day to be sufficient to accomplish this.[8] For athletes between 150 and 200 pounds, this works out to be 96 to 128 grams per day of protein. Most athletes admit they consume protein in amounts beyond the highest recommended intake levels of between 1.7 and 2.0 grams/kg/day.[9,10] There's no data to support any increased benefit in doing so.

In all actuality, the evidence points to the opposite as a number of harmful health effects develop when the body increases in size. NFL linemen, who are considered to be some of the largest athletes in the world, have increased risks of cardiovascular disease and metabolic syndrome compared to their fellow teammates.[11] Larger athletes also have a shorter lifespan due to their increased body weight, confirming once again that more is not always better.[12]

True protein deficiencies are rare and are usually only seen in developing countries where famine and malnutrition are more prevalent. A small segment of the population has a genetic disorder prohibiting them from producing certain proteins. Protein C and S deficiencies are such conditions. They are inherited disorders, which are not related to diet.[13]

Cachexia is another medical disorder unrelated to diet. It results in an increase in protein breakdown and a depletion of skeletal muscle due to a chronic, systemic inflammatory response occurring in the body.[14] It's typically associated with chronic infections or malignant conditions. You've probably seen this in advanced cancer patients as they "waste" away toward the end of their life. Unfortunately, cachexia cannot be reversed by consuming more dietary protein or drinking protein supplements.[15]

Kwashiorkor and Marasmus are the common dietary-related protein deficiencies most people think about when envisioning a lack of protein.[16] An image of a malnourished child, who is all skin and bones, is the classic portrayal for these disorders. Kwashiorkor and Marasmus typically affect children in developing countries where food sources are scarce. They rarely occur in countries like the United States.

Protein is a readily available nutrient found in more than just burgers, chicken breasts, and chili dogs. To most people's surprise many plant-based foods contain significant amounts of protein. Provided below is a chart comparing the amount of protein in various plant and animal foods. Notice how green vegetables contain just as much protein on a calorie per calorie basis as beef and chicken.

There has been considerable debate over the quality of protein and whether or not plant foods contain as high a quality of protein as animal foods. When the term *quality* is used to describe protein, it is in reference to the amino acid composition of protein. There are twenty different amino acids that can be used to form a protein, and eight of these are considered essential.[17] Essential amino acids must be obtained from the diet. The body cannot make them on its own.

> Green vegetables contain just as much protein on a calorie per calorie basis as beef and chicken.

Many people mistakenly believe only meat and dairy provide all the essential amino acids packaged into one source, therefore making them of a higher quality protein than plant foods. They argue that a diet comprised

Food Item	Protein (grams per 100 calories)
Chicken breast, meat and skin, raw	12
Hamburger, 90% lean ground beef, raw	11
Skim milk	10
Egg	9
Cheddar cheese	6
Spinach	12
Broccoli, florets	11
Asparagus	11
Black beans, cooked	7
Kale	6

Source: USDA National Nutrient Database for Standard Reference via www.NutritionData.com, Accessed Nov 10th, 2011.

only of plant-based foods is somehow deficient in one or more essential amino acids. This is not true.

In an article published in 2002 in the journal *Circulation,* Dr. John McDougall stated otherwise: "A careful look at the founding scientific research and some simple math prove it is impossible to design an amino acid deficient diet based on the amounts of unprocessed starches and vegetables sufficient to meet the calorie needs of humans. Furthermore, mixing foods to make a complementary amino acid composition is unnecessary."[18]

The clever marketing tactics used in our culture to promote excessive protein consumption has accomplished its goal. Hundreds of millions of people now believe a diet lacking large amounts of animal protein or protein in general will result in undesirable effects to one's health. The exact opposite is true. Plant-based proteins are not associated with the same chronic diseases animal-based proteins are associated with. Instead, they're filled with tens of thousands of disease-fighting antioxidants and phytochemicals crucial for optimal health and disease prevention, which are completely absent in animal-based foods. Getting enough protein has never been the problem in America. Getting the right kind has.

No Dairy Products? How Do You Get Your Calcium?

Ever since we were old enough to watch a television ad, we've been taught to associate healthy bones with black-and-white dairy cows. After all, how is one supposed to grow up big and strong if a glass of milk isn't part of a healthy breakfast or cheese isn't included in salads and sandwiches? This is exactly how I grew up, and the notion that enough calcium was available in anything other than dairy products was a foreign concept to me. It sounded absolutely absurd to be honest. I'm sure you may even agree.

The significance of getting enough calcium to maintain healthy growth and development is legitimate. Calcium is not only important for bone health but also plays a crucial role in many other processes in the body. It's required for normal blood clotting, maintaining a healthy heartbeat, sending and receiving nerve signals, proper muscle movement, and the release of certain hormones in the body.[19-21] Without calcium we'd be in dire straits.

How much calcium is needed to meet our body's needs is, once again, another topic of confusion for the general public. Doctors are even misled on this subject. This is largely due to the marketing efforts of the dairy industry. Their only motives are to increase profits not look out for the health of the general population.

In 2010, the Institute of Medicine (IOM) published the most recent recommendations for calcium intake levels.[22] These levels are the gold standard by which the medical and nutritional communities currently base their practices. The IOM recommends male adults between the ages of 19 and 70 years old consume a minimum of 1,000 mg/day of calcium and at least 1,200 mg/day for those over the age of 70. Females between the ages of 19 and 50 years of age should consume 1,000 mg/day according to the IOM. After 50 years of age females are supposed to consume 1,200 mg/day of calcium. The IOM developed their calcium recommendations by using data from the study referenced in the next paragraph.

In 2007 the *American Journal of Clinical Nutrition* reviewed data on calcium balance from a total of nineteen different studies spanning a twenty-year period.[23] Researchers concluded that a total of 741 mg/day of calcium was needed to achieve adequate calcium balance in healthy individuals regardless of age or sex. The IOM, however, based their calcium recommendations not by choosing the average requirement of 741 mg/day of calcium, but rather by choosing the upper limit of 1,035 mg/day of calcium and then rounding up or down based on the age and/or sex of the patient.

The IOM also failed to take into account comments made later in this study stating "that individuals with low, but nutritionally adequate, intakes of sodium and protein may have calcium requirements as low as 500 mg/day." Low, but nutritionally adequate, intakes of sodium and protein is the very definition of a whole foods, plant-based diet. Those who follow a whole foods, plant-based lifestyle do not overconsume protein or sodium like those on the Standard American Diet of beef, chicken, pork, dairy, eggs, cheese, and processed foods. For them, achieving calcium requirements of 500 mg/day is not an issue.

For those on a typical Western diet there are a few dietary factors that have been shown to increase calcium losses from the body. These include high intakes of sodium, caffeine, and phosphorus.[24-26] These substances are typically found in beverages such as energy drinks, soda pop, and coffee. They're also found in canned foods, snacks, and animal products. These are all nutrient-deficient foods that do not meet the description of a diet with "low, but nutritionally adequate, intakes of sodium and protein," as mentioned in the previous study.

This makes it clear that diets of animal-based and processed foods require higher amounts of calcium intake to counter the imbalances created by these very foods. You can avoid having to constantly replace such large amounts of calcium in the body by enjoying the benefits of a whole foods, plant-based lifestyle and staying away from meat and dairy entirely.

To many people's surprise, calcium is abundant in a number of different plant foods including dark leafy greens, legumes, and whole grains as shown in the chart below. It's also better absorbed by the body when obtained from green vegetables such as green beans, broccoli, bok choy, and kale than it is from cow's milk.[27,28] One exception seems to be vegetables with high oxalate content such as spinach. Oxalates can bind to calcium interfering with its absorption.[29] This doesn't mean you don't acquire any calcium from spinach, nor does it mean you should avoid spinach. Spinach is a healthy food. It only serves as a reminder for us to include a variety of whole, plant-based foods as part of the overall diet.

Calcium Content in Various Foods			
Animal-based foods	Calcium content (mg)	**Plant-based foods**	Calcium content (mg)
Yogurt (vanilla, low fat) 8 oz container, 1 cup	388	Soy milk (fortified), 1 cup	299
Sardines, Atlantic (canned) 1 can	351	Collard greens (cooked), 1 cup	266
Cow's milk (skim), 1 cup	306	Almond milk (unsweetened), 1 cup	200
Cow's milk (2%), 1 cup	286	Navy beans (cooked), 1 cup	126
Cow's milk (whole), 1 cup	276	Okra (cooked), 1 cup	123
Swiss cheese, 1 slice	221	Amaranth grain (cooked), 1 cup	116
Cheddar cheese, 1 slice	202	Swiss Chard (cooked), 1 cup	101
Ice cream, vanilla 1 cup	169	Kale (raw), 1 cup	91
Fish, Atlantic herring 1 fillet	106	Chickpeas (cooked), 1 cup	80
Sour cream, 2 oz	80	Almonds, 1 oz	74
Salmon, wild Atlantic 1 fillet	46	Orange, Florida	65
Cream, half & half, 1 oz	31	Broccoli (cooked), 1 cup	62
Egg, hardboiled	25	Spinach (raw), 1 cup	30

Source: USDA National Nutrient Database for Standard Reference via www.NutritionData.com, Accessed November 20th, 2011.

Are Vegetarians Sick and Malnourished?

A common belief is that all vegetarians are sick, malnourished, and weak. It's understandable why others might think so. The stereotypical image that comes to mind of a vegetarian or vegan is a small-framed hippie who wears quirky, colorful clothing and sprouts a scraggly beard over pale skin. However, this certainly wouldn't be enough to qualify them as being sick or malnourished. It also doesn't mean there aren't people who resemble this same depiction who consume a Standard American Diet.

Remember the saying, "Don't judge a book by its cover." Just because something may appear one way on the outside doesn't mean it's true when you start peeling away the layers to see what it looks like on the inside. You'd be surprised at how many "average" looking people follow a plant-based lifestyle.

The information presented in this book isn't about labeling yourself a vegan or vegetarian, although you may technically end up as one after reading it. Instead, it's about helping you become the best you can be. The "v" words only focus on what's left out of the diet and not what's incorporated into the diet. These labels were not designed to put optimal health at center stage. This is what makes plant-based living unique. It focuses on achieving optimal health, allowing for both a longer and healthier life.

The idea that vegans (people who consume no meat, dairy, or eggs) and vegetarians (people who forgo meat but may still consume dairy and eggs) are not as healthy as nonvegetarians holds some truth to it when such individuals don't structure their diet properly.[30] I know of several people who are vegetarian or vegan and in poor health because they are "junk food" eaters. They may not consume meat or dairy products, but they consume a large amount of nutrient-deficient junk foods that are highly refined and processed. Examples include Oreo cookies, Nature Valley® Peanut Butter Crunchy Granola Bars, and Kellogg's Special K® Protein Plus cereal, all of which are vegan, but these foods put vegans and vegetarians at risk for the same chronic diseases everyone else gets in America.

Vegetarians and vegans may have chosen to eat this way for ethical or environmental reasons. If this is the case, then I commend them for their efforts and appreciate their willingness to do something to make the world a better place. I also care about them as a person though and want them to experience the health benefits of eating a nutritionally optimal diet. That way they can continue to be at their best and make a positive impact on the world around them for an even longer time.

The truth of the matter is this: adopting a plant-based lifestyle is the best thing you can do for your health. The cultures around the world that have the lowest rates of chronic diseases thrive off a foundation of nutrient-dense, plant-based, whole foods. Vegetables, fruits, legumes, and whole grains are staples in their diet. Healthy lives abound from the residents of Japan, to the islanders of Papua New Guinea, to the citizens of India as long as they stick to their traditional plant-based foods.

But if they adopt rich Western food, they soon develop debilitating Western diseases. This is quite typical with younger generations of these cultures. The older generations tend to flourish well into their eighties and nineties, if not past 100 years old. One group of people in particular, the residents of Okinawa, are a shining example of longevity.

Okinawa is a group of islands in the southernmost portion of Japan—home to the greatest concentration of healthy, long-living individuals on the face of the planet. Numerous studies have been conducted to figure out how so many of these residents are able to live such vibrant, active lives with little to no signs of chronic illness. Their secrets lie with getting back to the basics.

Okinawans remain physically active throughout their life, practice caloric restriction, and eat a traditional diet comprised heavily of vegetables (orange-yellow root vegetables and dark leafy greens), fruit, legumes (mostly soy), low glycemic grains, and only small amounts of fish or other animal products.[31] There's no such thing as Burger King, Wonder Bread, or even vegan hot dogs in their diets. If there were, Okinawans certainly wouldn't be getting the recognition they've gotten for years about their health and longevity. Scientists and health experts around the world rave about them.

Isn't Going Plant-Based Boring and Expensive?

One of the many reasons people say they can't go plant-based is because it's too expensive or too boring. I say those are great excuses to continue to eat the same two things (animal-based and processed foods) comprised of the same three ingredients (fat, sugar, and salt) for the rest of your life. Your hard-earned dollars and, more importantly, your overall health will continue to be at the mercy of the medical and pharmaceutical industries if you choose to keep living this way.

Switching to a plant-based lifestyle can be expensive, and it can also be boring *if* you let it be. Just like anything in life, the situation is what you make of it. Ever go to dinner and a movie? This can be expensive and boring depending on how pricey the restaurant is and which movie you choose. On the other hand, you could have a fabulous home-cooked dinner and rent an Academy Award–winning blockbuster for a fraction of the cost if you choose to do so.

The same goes for plant-based nutrition. Some produce items are expensive, especially if you buy them from higher-end grocery stores or specialty health food stores. These same items can often cost 25 to 50 percent less at a local farmers' market or fruit and vegetable stand. Even your local grocer may have these same items for bargain prices in their weekly sales ad.

Frozen fruits and vegetables are another great option for staying healthy and saving money. You can also buy certain items in bulk, such as dried beans, canned goods, and nuts and seeds. Doing so will help you pay a much lower price without sacrificing quality. These items are typically shelf stable for several weeks or even months making them ideal items to stock up on especially when on sale.

As for the boring part, this is another misnomer about plant-based nutrition. Several studies and surveys attest to how widely accepted plant-based diets can be. One study followed just under 100 diabetics for 74 weeks.[32] Half the group was given the American Diabetes Association (ADA) diet and the other half consumed 100 percent of their calories from low-fat, plant-based foods. The plant-based group had just as high an acceptance rate as the ADA group but also experienced a greater reduction in cravings for fatty foods—an added bonus.

Another study compared two groups of women. One group was put on the National Cholesterol Education Program (NCEP) diet and the other on a low-fat, plant-based regimen.[33] The plant-based group had high acceptability ratings similar to the NCEP group but also experienced less constraint with dietary requirements. This is likely due to the absence of calorie counting or portion control, which is not required when following a plant-based lifestyle. The NCEP participants also stated the continuation of their new diet long term would be more difficult to sustain than their previous diet. This is typical of how most people feel on diet programs.

More support for the likability of plant-based eating comes in the form of a survey conducted in 2011.[34] In this survey, over 2,000 individuals who currently followed a plant-based lifestyle were asked if they enjoy the food they eat. An overwhelming 96.7 percent said yes. What's more, 94.4 percent said they planned on eating this way for the rest of their lives. People don't typically continue eating the same way long term if they find it boring. This survey proves once again how satisfying plant-based living can be.

As a final note, I'd like to share with you a couple of invaluable resources I've come across that do wonders for keeping a healthy variety of flavor in your diet, while at the same time keeping your monthly grocery bill under control. Jeff Novick, RD, has produced a series of instructional videos called *Jeff Novick's Fast Food*. His recipes are healthy, simple to make, take less than ten to fifteen minutes to prepare, and can all be done at a cost of less than $5 a day. Another resource is from long-distance runner Ellen Jaffe Jones. Her book *Eat Vegan on $4 a Day* has numerous whole foods, plant-based recipes to choose from that won't break the bank. These outstanding items make plant-based living easy, inexpensive, delicious, and irresistible!

Isn't a Plant-Based Lifestyle Safe for Adults but Not Children?

Contrary to popular belief, children do not need to eat animal-based foods to grow up strong and healthy. The more meat, dairy, and sugary foods a child eats, the higher the risk of becoming overweight.[35,36] These poor dietary habits have been shown to increase the risk of cancer and cardiovascular disease in later adult years.[37,38]

The opposite holds true for children who grow up consuming mainly plant-based foods. By avoiding meat, these children are leaner and much less likely to become overweight as they reach adolescence.[39] These favorable eating habits also serve to lessen the risk of obesity-related diseases as the child grows older.

Dr. Joel Fuhrman, author of *Disease-Proof Your Child*, sums it up best as he speaks about the link between childhood nutritional patterns and overall health: "Over the past two decades convincing evidence has emerged which links autoimmune illnesses, such as Crohn's Disease, lupus and later-life cancers with precise dietary factors from the first ten years of life ... we now know what factors help to create an environment in our bodies which is favorable for cancers to surface later in life, and we understand the precise dietary factors that can prevent cancer in our child's future ... Humans, like other primates, are designed to consume a diet predominating in natural plant foods ... Fresh fruits, vegetables, beans, raw nuts and seeds should form the foundation of normal nutrition."[40]

Health doesn't start at the age of eighteen. It starts before you're even born. Once weaned off mother's breast milk, children thrive on an assortment of plant-based, whole foods. Not only does this ensure the avoidance of childhood obesity but also protects against an onslaught of chronic diseases later in life. No parent would ever provide their children with cigarettes knowing the health risks associated with them. Similar health risks await millions of children being fed a typical Western diet. Knowledge is power. Perhaps it's time to rethink what ends up on the dinner table in your family home. After all, aren't your kids worth it?

Move It or Lose It—
The Benefits of Exercising

*"A vigorous five-mile walk will do more good for
an unhappy but otherwise healthy adult than all
the medicine and psychology in the world."*
—PAUL DUDLEY WHITE

Exercise and health are like two peas in a pod. They go hand in hand. The more you exercise, the more health benefits you get. The more health benefits you get, the more you feel like exercising. But how much exercise do you need? Should you join a gym? What types of exercises should you be doing?

These are all common questions people have. It can be tough to sort through all of them too, especially with the overwhelming number of choices today. If you followed everyone's advice, you'd have three different gym memberships, every conceivable piece of exercise equipment known to man, and a full-time personal trainer to boot. It doesn't have to be this complicated though.

First, I want to remind you that following a lifestyle consisting almost entirely, if not 100 percent, of plant-based, whole foods trumps everything else when it comes to health and longevity. Without a strong foundation of healthy, wholesome foods in your everyday diet, you can exercise until you're blue in the face and still end up in poor health. Excellent health is attained through healthy eating habits; taking it to the next level is achieved through getting consistent amounts of regular exercise.

The Godfather of Fitness

One of his most famous lines was, "I can't die, it would ruin my image."[1] Better known as the Godfather of Fitness, Jack LaLanne was one of the most youthful and vivacious human beings ever to walk the face of the planet. He worked out two hours every day and continued these workouts well into his nineties, up until the age of ninety-six when he sadly died of severe pneumonia. The chance of his image being ruined, however, is as improbable as the sun not rising each day.

Jack was light years ahead of his time. He was using fitness and nutrition as his primary means of achieving optimal health long before it became popular in today's culture. This wasn't always the case in his life though. In his earlier years when he was a young boy, Jack was a "sugaraholic" and "junk food junkie," as he described it. This all changed at the age of fifteen when he heard the famous nutritionist Paul Bragg give a lecture on how eating right and exercising could help achieve amazing health results. From that point forward Jack was hooked. He immediately set aside the sugar-laden junk food and headed to the local YMCA to test out their weights.

Jack would soon epitomize what it meant to be the ultimate health icon. He became America's leading fitness guru starting in the mid-1930s. He opened the nation's first modern health spa in 1936 and started promoting working out and lifting weights long before doctors of his time bought into his methodology.

He was met with fierce resistance from mainstream medicine as he described it, "People thought I was a charlatan and a nut. The doctors were against me—they said that working out with weights would give people heart attacks and they would lose their sex drive. Women would look like men and even varsity coaches predicted that their athletes would get muscle bound and banned them from lifting weights. I had to give these athletes keys so they could come in at night and work out in my gym."

We can thank Jack LaLanne for paving the way for what science would soon come to prove over the second half of the twentieth century, that leading an active lifestyle has many profound health benefits. Jack was not only the first to get athletes and women in the gym lifting weights and working out, but also the first to combine weight training and nutrition.

Jack became famous for juicing fresh fruits and vegetables as part of his daily diet and even developed his own line of juicing machines that continue to be sold today. His motto when it came to food was, "If man makes it, don't eat it."

The fitness world will forever be indebted to Jack's contributions and accomplishments and so will the fields of science and medicine. We can take many lessons from the Godfather of Fitness. You're about to find out what those are next.

Everyday Habits, Extraordinary Results, and Fun In Between

You don't have to work out two hours a day and push yourself to the limit like Jack LaLanne to reap the rewards of exercise. If you choose to do so, there's certainly nothing wrong with that. It will only increase the degree of health benefits you see, both physically and mentally, as a result of your efforts. This has been proven in the scientific literature time and time again as the rates of all-cause mortality go down when the amount of regular physical activity goes up in an individual's life. As little as thirty minutes a day, five days a week of moderate intensity activity can reduce your overall risk of death by 19 percent.[2] This increases to a 24 percent reduction when an individual engages in an hour of exercise each day.

Regular amounts of exercise reduce the risk of numerous chronic diseases such as cardiovascular disease, diabetes, cancer, osteoporosis, obesity, and depression. The following are just a few of the examples of how regular physical activity accomplishes this:[3]

- Lowers blood pressure
- Reduces triglyceride levels
- Increases HDL "good" cholesterol levels
- Normalizes blood glucose levels and increases insulin sensitivity
- Reduces systemic inflammation
- Decreases the risk of blood clots
- Improves coronary blood flow
- Reduces abdominal fat
- Enhances endothelial function
- Reduces stress, anxiety, and depression
- Increases metabolism
- Boosts the immune system
- Strengthens bones by increasing bone mineral density

Another interesting fact about exercise has to do with its effect on cellular aging. Our cells make us who we are. We couldn't function without them, nor would we want to. They serve as the building blocks for our tissues, organs, and systems found throughout our entire body. The unique thing about our cells is they have the ability to replicate and divide to form new cells, and thus replace older existing cells worn out from days, months, or even years of wear and tear.

Our cells rely completely and totally on our DNA to carry out this process. Our genetic code, therefore, provides the "blueprint" for cell division and, ultimately, life itself. When our DNA becomes damaged, the new cells generated are not always as perfect as previous versions were. Hence, the aging process. Our heart may not beat as strong, our skin becomes wrinkled, and we have a hard time keeping up with life like we used to. Whatever it is, we're getting older.

There's a catch to this whole aging process though. The catch is that while chronological aging (time elapsed since birth) is inevitable, biological aging (physiological breakdown of the body) is not, or at the very least it can be delayed. We can control how fast our body ages depending on how we choose to live our life. This is accomplished by protecting or enhancing the length of our telomeres.[4]

> **We can control how fast our body ages depending on how we choose to live our life.**

Telomeres are found at the very end of DNA strands and act as a protective barrier by preventing ensuing damage to the DNA itself. Think of them like the hard plastic protectors at the ends of a shoestring. If the plastic protectors start to wear down, they eventually fall off and the shoestring starts to fray and fall apart. The same holds true for our DNA strands. They need their plastic protectors (telomeres) at the end of their double helix in order to stay intact keeping them from "fraying" or unraveling. This will ensure that a workable blueprint is available for healthy cellular replication. So how do we protect our telomeres?

One of the most well-researched items to date on this subject has to do with exercise. Moderate regular physical activity has been shown to provide the greatest protection against shortened telomere length in individuals maintaining an exercise program for five or more years.[5] On the other hand short-term physical activity, a sedentary lifestyle, and overtraining (two hours per day or more of high-intensity workouts) have all been linked to shorter telomere lengths. The take home message from this is if you want to live longer and age slower, then a regular moderate exercise program is a must. You'll feel better, look younger, and have more energy resulting in a win/win/win situation.

Before you begin any exercise program, it's important to talk to your doctor to get the all clear. This will ensure you won't worsen any current medical condition you may have or increase your risk of injury by trying to do too much too fast. Once you receive the all clear, then make it a priority to get regular physical exercise. Make an appointment with yourself if you have to so there are no excuses holding you back. You can always start out slowly and build your way up to where you need to be.

It's important to pick activities you enjoy. After all, if you choose to join a runner's club but hate running, then chances are you're never going to stick with it. On the other hand, if you love bicycling, then join a cycling club or search for new trails close by to ride. The activity you choose doesn't have to be extravagant. Whether it's as simple as gardening or as relaxing as a basic walk around the neighborhood, just do something and make sure you're having fun while doing it. If you're up for a bigger challenge, then try to make the following four types of exercises part of your normal routine. You'll achieve optimal fitness results by doing so.

Four Main Types of Exercise

Developing a great overall workout program, according to the American College of Sports Medicine (ACSM), should always focus on four categories of exercises—flexibility, neuromotor, strength, and cardiorespiratory training.[6] Each one has its own unique role in promoting optimal health while working out different parts of the body.

It's always a good idea to have a personal trainer or someone with similar expertise to get you started with each type of exercise. This way you'll learn the correct techniques and avoid injuries as well as increase your overall results.

Flexibility Training (Stretching, Range of Motion)

Flexibility training is all about stretching and loosening up those knotted muscles. As part of a general warm-up routine, stretching can decrease the risk of muscle strains before participating in sporting events.[7] It's also beneficial if you don't compete in sports, as it can significantly increase your range of motion in joints and muscles throughout your body.[8] Either way it's important to include flexibility training as part of your comprehensive workout routine.

According to the ACSM, strive to get at least two days per week of this type of training. Even as little as ten to fifteen minutes per session can be beneficial. It's also the perfect type of exercise to pick if you need help building up to more intense workouts but cannot physically handle more vigorous forms of exercising right away.

Some excellent ways to liven up flexibility training, besides everyday stretching, is to take a yoga or Pilates class. Both will provide a gentle challenge, and it's a fantastic way to meet other people. You can also try Tai chi, which is based on the ancient Chinese practice of slow, gentle exercises and stretches to keep the body moving from one posture to the next. Tai chi has its roots in martial arts and is self-paced, noncompetitive, and relaxing. It's a wonderful way to reduce stress.

Neuromotor Exercise Training

Neuromotor training may be an unfamiliar term to many, but it's not as mysterious as it sounds. All it means is to engage in exercises that improve balance, coordination, gait, and agility. It's what keeps athletes quick and nimble and also what helps elderly people improve their stability and balance, decreasing their risk of falls.[9,10] The ACSM recommends incorporating neuromotor training into your exercise regimen a total of two to three days per week with sessions lasting twenty to thirty minutes each.

One of the best ways to do this is Tai chi. Tai chi has been well studied as a form of neuromotor training and has proven benefits in improving balance, agility, motor control, and proprioception (your sense of balance in time and space).[11] You could also try yoga or plyometrics as another form of neuromotor training. One last option is the practice of Qigong. Qigong is another exercise with traditional Chinese roots. It even dates back before Tai chi. Qigong is defined as a combination of breathing, fluid movements, and meditation all in one. It not only improves balance and coordination but also helps reduce the incidence of depression and anxiety.[12]

Strength Training (Resistance Exercises)

Strength training, or resistance training, is the activity most people envision when they think of someone working out at the gym. It's the barbell curls, bench presses, and dumbbell lunges that work to tone and strengthen the major muscle groups in the body.[13] If you love the gym, then you'll love this type of exercising, but that doesn't mean you have to become the next world champion bodybuilder to partake in this activity. It also doesn't mean you have to spend hours each day pumping iron.

Strength training can be done from the comfort of your own home with no equipment at all if you prefer. Push-ups and sit-ups are excellent ways to strengthen muscles. You can use resistance bands or purchase an inexpensive set of dumbbells to use at home. Whatever works for you is perfectly fine as long as you're strengthening the major muscle groups of the body.

The benefits of strength training go far beyond just building bigger and stronger muscles. These exercises have shown benefits in overall health by improving metabolic functioning and reducing the risk of cardiovascular disease and diabetes.[14] Resistance training helps generate more mitochondria (in muscle fibers) leading to higher energy levels.[15] Finally, impact or resistance exercises show a clear benefit in increasing bone density and reducing the risk of osteoporosis in both men and women.[16]

The ACSM recommends strength training two to three days per week and targeting all the major muscle groups throughout the week. You can do this by switching the target areas on different days. For example, you could work out legs the first day, back and biceps the next, and chest, shoulder, and triceps the final day of the week.

Cardiorespiratory Training (Aerobic Exercise)

Cardiorespiratory training is more commonly referred to as "cardio" or aerobic exercising. The goal of this exercise is to improve the efficiency of the heart, lungs, and blood vessels. This is done by exercising to your age-specific target heart rate for a specified amount of time. The ACSM recommends most adults engage in moderate intensity aerobic exercise for thirty minutes per day, five days a week OR vigorous-intensity aerobic exercise for twenty minutes per day, three days per week.

This can be accomplished by exercising at 60 to 90 percent of your maximum heart rate (HRmax), which is determined by using either one of the following equations calculated using your age:[17]

Karvonen Equation	Tanaka Equation
HRmax = 220 - age	HRmax = 208 - (0.7 x age)

Both equations achieved similar results, according to a study in 2008, when predicting actual measured maximum heart rates for healthy adults during a controlled exercise program.[18] If you would rather keep things simple, then just know you've reached your target heart rate zone if you feel uncomfortable talking while trying to breathe normally during your workout session.

Participating in an aerobic workout program comes along with a host of health benefits. In addition to lowering blood pressure and cholesterol levels, it also reduces overall mortality from coronary artery disease, helps with weight loss efforts, reduces anxiety and depression, and improves the management of diabetes, pregnancy, and aging.[19] Moreover, aerobic exercise may dramatically benefit the sleeping habits of those who routinely include cardio in their workout regimen. Studies show that individuals who are physically active average 1.25 hours more sleep per night than those who are not active. These individuals experience a much higher quality of sleep too.[20]

Considering all the wonderful health benefits you get for spending a mere 1.5 percent of your total time each week on cardiorespiratory workouts, it's definitely worth the effort to get off the couch and get moving. Go bicycling, jogging, swimming, or grab that old tennis racket and drag a friend to your local tennis courts. Do something to stay active and make sure it's something you enjoy so you continue to do it for many years to come.

Excuses, Excuses, Excuses—Don't Be Your Own Enabler

I'll be the first to admit that I hate exercising. I wasn't born with a burning desire to take a five-mile joy run every day or participate in a grueling class of kickboxing three times a week. I was never a star athlete when growing up and would much rather watch a sporting event than compete in one. If I had my way I would've created the human body to thrive by exercising less instead of more, but unfortunately this isn't the case. Our bodies need exercise whether we like it or not.

There is one thing, however, that I do love about exercise. I love how it makes me feel after I'm done. I love the extra energy I get throughout the day, the better sleep I get at night, and the increased mental clarity that comes along with it. Exercise does wonders in that respect for me. It can do the same for you.

We will always make excuses for not having enough time or being completely exhausted or the kids needing you to do something for them, but these are just that—excuses! There are only two kinds of people in this world when it comes to not exercising on a regular basis—sick people and soon-to-be sick people. It would be three types of people, but dead people don't count.

Get up, get out, and start moving your body. If you can only handle five minutes of exercise, then do five minutes of exercise. The next time try increasing it to six minutes. It may not always be fun especially in the beginning. You may have a little voice inside your head that keeps telling you to stop because you can't possibly go any further. If this happens then do what I do and tell yourself, "Self, I'll be damned if some imaginary little voice is going to determine what I can and cannot do. It's my turn to run the show. Silence!" I can't tell you how many times this has enabled me to get another thirty seconds or more out of my workout. Before you know it, you'll be up to thirty or even sixty minutes of continuous exercise in one workout session. I know you have it within you to make it happen. You and your body deserve nothing less than your best!

Supplement Wisely

"Adam and Eve ate the first vitamins,
including the package."

—E.R. SQUIBB

Before kids across America head off to school each day, many will heed the call of their parents as they head out the door, "Did you take your vitamins?" Vitamins and other supplements are as commonplace in American households as prescription drugs. We love to take our pills, and it shows by how much money is spent on dietary supplements. An article in *Time* magazine in 2011 stated that America spends $28 billion a year on dietary supplements, $5 billion more than is spent on gym memberships.[1]

While private investors and other conglomerates spend billions each year in research and development hoping to formulate the next "miracle pill," the question we should be asking ourselves is whether any of these supplements actually work. If so, which ones do and which ones are a waste of our money? Finally, are there any downsides to taking supplements?

As a practicing pharmacist, I am extremely confident when saying there are no "miracle pills" out there. I've never seen one to date and highly doubt that I, nor anybody else, ever will during the course of my lifetime.

177

The harder the human race works to isolate or synthesize individual compounds by putting them into pill form, the more problems we seem to create by doing so. Every day we read reports of how this vitamin or that vitamin is causing more harm than good.

Just because an item is available over-the-counter (OTC) doesn't mean it's free of possible side effects. In fact, OTC products can be just as dangerous, if not more so, than prescription drugs. Unlike prescription drugs, the FDA has to actually prove supplements are unsafe before taking any action against the manufacturers

> OTC products can be just as dangerous, if not more so, than prescription drugs.

who make them.[2] This is the complete opposite from the position taken against drug manufacturers who are required to prove both safety and efficacy of their products before being allowed to sell them. We all know how well that's turned out. Prescription medications are littered with adverse effects.

Although some people taking dietary supplements may see some benefits, it's important to note these benefits are only short term, acting as a quick fix for a much larger problem. Heart disease, diabetes, autoimmune disorders, and other degenerative diseases are not going to reverse course after you pop a handful of vitamins every morning. There are few legitimate uses for a small number of select vitamins and supplements, which I will go over in this chapter, but the vast majority of them are worthless. I will also address a number of major concerns about some commonly consumed supplements.

A Multivitamin a Day?

Multivitamins are the most widely used of all supplements. Over 40 percent of adults in the United States reported using multivitamins according to the latest survey from the National Center for Health Statistics.[3] If you ask someone why they take a multivitamin, they would surely give you an answer similar to this: "To make up for whatever vitamins and minerals I don't get in my diet. I figure the more the better and a multivitamin can't hurt me."

It turns out a multivitamin *can* hurt you. Reports from various medical journals have revealed the hidden truth about the safety and efficacy of multivitamin supplementation. The *Archives of Internal Medicine* analyzed data from the Iowa Women's Health Study on the use of various dietary supplements in more than 38,000 women over an eighteen-year period.

Researchers reported an increased risk in overall mortality with the use of multivitamins, vitamin B6, folic acid, iron, magnesium, zinc, and copper compared to those women not taking the supplements.[4]

In 2010, the *American Journal of Clinical Nutrition* published their findings on the link between multivitamin use and breast cancer.[5] Researchers followed over 35,000 cancer-free women for a period of nine and a half years. Users of multivitamin supplements showed a 19 percent overall increased risk of developing breast cancer despite being leaner in body size, on average, than nonusers. This is alarming because we already know the risk of breast cancer increases as obesity rates increase in women.[6] This study now shows the use of multivitamin supplements add to this risk of developing breast cancer even in non-obese women.

The news isn't much better for men, as the *Journal of Clinical Oncology* points out in a published report on the use of vitamin and mineral supplementation in cancer survivors. The 2010 review states, "Excess consumption of one or a combination of components in a multivitamin/ multi-mineral may accelerate cancer progression and increase fatality" for men suffering from prostate cancer.[7] These findings were similar to a 2007 report in the *Journal of the National Cancer Institute*. In this report, men taking multivitamins on a regular basis saw no benefit in terms of prostate cancer risk and actually experienced an increased risk of advanced and fatal cases of prostate cancer when taking more than one multivitamin supplement per day.[8]

What's going on here? Isn't getting more vitamins and minerals in our body supposed to be beneficial? The answer to this question is a resounding yes *if* the vitamins and minerals are obtained from their natural sources— plant-based, whole foods.

Investigators from the United Kingdom acknowledge this fact as they report suboptimal intakes of micronutrients increase the risk of diseases such as cancer and cardiovascular disease.[9] They go on to say that randomized trials of using vitamin and mineral supplements in people with chronic diseases failed to show any clinical improvements in their conditions. Investigators recommended instead that future studies concentrate on using whole, plant-based foods (fruits and vegetables) to produce any meaningful outcomes in individuals with chronic illnesses.

A 2008 article in the *American Journal of Public Health* reported similar views on the use of multivitamins in older adults. In this report, authors challenged the suggestion of Congress to require multivitamin supplementation in elderly patients as an addition to meals as part of the Older Americans Act (OAA) Nutrition Program.[10] The authors state:

"Multivitamin-mineral supplements are not a quick fix for poor diets ... there is insufficient evidence of their benefits and safety. The program's limited funds and efforts should instead be directed to nutrient-dense healthy meals."

The researchers are correct. Human beings have never, and will never, be able to replicate all the goodness found in healthy, wholesome foods. There are literally hundreds of thousands of vitamins, minerals, and phytochemicals contained within these foods, some of which have yet to be discovered. These phytonutrients are crucial in achieving an optimal state of health.

To think a scientist and research lab can duplicate the work of nature in the form of a pill is like expecting a financial advisor to put together a flawless investment portfolio that never loses money, not even on a daily basis, for a financially driven venture capitalist. No one can perfect an outcome or a process based on information they don't have, especially when doing so is affected by an infinite number of interconnected variables over which there is no control.

Like world financial markets and global economies, the nutritional components of food are so complex with how they interact with each other it's virtually impossible to understand this on a human level. This is why the wisest decisions are often made in accordance with historical perspective. History tells us food is far superior to multivitamin supplements when supplying the nutrients we need for health and longevity. We should not expect anything else by cheating Mother Nature.

Concerns with Individual Supplements

Perhaps the best way to understand why multivitamins pose more of a risk to one's health than a benefit is by looking at the effect of individual vitamins and minerals contained within these formulations.

Vitamin E

Long touted for its benefits in preventing cardiovascular disease and cancer, vitamin E showed no such benefit after regular supplementation of 600 IU every other day in approximately 40,000 women who were followed for over a decade, according to a study in the *Journal of the American Medical Association (JAMA)*.[11] Data from this same group of women showed no benefit in vitamin E protecting against type 2 diabetes.[12]

Males supplementing with vitamin E actually experienced health-related consequences. An increased risk in hemorrhagic strokes, along with a significant increase in prostate cancer, was seen in healthy men taking 400 IU per day of vitamin E.[13,14] High dose vitamin E supplements have also been linked to higher overall mortality rates.[15] This may be due to the fact that synthetic versions of vitamin E used in supplements have a different chemical makeup than the natural forms of vitamin E found in food.

Vitamin E from whole food sources (nuts, seeds, dark leafy greens) has never been linked to any adverse effects and is therefore the preferred way to obtain this nutrient.[16]

Vitamin A and Carotenoids

This group of vitamins is known for its role in vision and growth and in maintaining a healthy immune system.[17] Many have heard of beta-carotene, a carotenoid that is eventually converted into vitamin A by the body. When consumed in natural forms (fruits and vegetables), carotenoids are beneficial to health, but when taken in supplement form, the opposite tends to prevail.

Studies have shown a higher incidence in lung cancer among smokers taking vitamin A supplements versus those who did not supplement.[18] Many different adverse effects have also been seen when taking high doses of vitamin A (≥ 75,000 IU/day) including headaches, vomiting, visual disturbances, enlargement of the spleen and liver, ascites (fluid build-up in the abdomen), dermatitis, anemia, and hyperglycemia.[19] In contrast, adverse effects are not seen when high amounts of carotenoids are consumed in the diet as whole, plant-based foods because the body is able to safely regulate how much of these carotenoids are converted to the active form of vitamin A (retinol) based on the body's needs.

Bone health is adversely affected by vitamin A supplementation. Women regularly taking vitamin A supplements have been shown to have a 40 percent increased risk in developing osteoporosis compared to those not supplementing.[20] The increase in bone fractures may be due to vitamin A reducing the ability of vitamin D to increase intestinal calcium absorption in the diet.[21]

Because of the deleterious effects of vitamin A supplementation, the Institute of Medicine does not recommend supplementing with vitamin A carotenoids and, instead, suggests increasing consumption of carotenoid-rich fruits and vegetables.[22]

Folic Acid

Folic acid is the synthetic version of folate, which is naturally found in foods such as dark leafy greens, beans, peas, nuts, and fruits.[23] It is most widely known for its ability to reduce neural tube birth defects when pregnant women either take folic acid supplements or increase folate consumption in their diets.[24] What's less widely known are the poor outcomes and other dangerous effects linked to taking folic acid supplements when used to treat diseases such as cardiovascular disease and cancer.

A 2010 meta-analysis, published in the *American Journal of Cardiology*, showed no benefit in reducing cardiovascular disease or stroke in those taking folic acid supplements despite the fact folic acid should have a homocysteine-lowering effect, which would, in theory, reduce the rates of these diseases.[25] In contrast, high dietary intakes of folate are associated with a reduced risk of mortality from stroke, coronary heart disease, and heart failure in individuals.[26]

One of the biggest concerns regarding folic acid is the increased risk in cancer seen when taking this supplement. A 2011 meta-analysis showed a 35 percent increased incidence in advanced colorectal tumors in those supplementing with folic acid over a three-year period or longer.[27] Another study showed an increased risk of prostate cancer in men supplementing with folic acid but a decreased risk in men consuming higher amounts of folate in their diet.[28]

The same correlation holds true for breast cancer risk in women. Data from the PLCO Cancer Screening trial indicated a 20 percent increased risk of breast cancer in women supplementing with 400 mcg or more per day of folic acid.[29] In contrast, an inverse relationship was seen between breast cancer occurrence and high dietary intake of folate in women.

Folic acid fortification of food or taken in supplement form can also mask the following medical conditions—anemia of vitamin B12 deficiency, leukemia, arthritis, bowel cancer, and ectopic pregnancies.[30] These effects are not seen when natural forms of folate are consumed from whole foods.

Omega-3 Fatty Acids

Omega-3 fatty acids are commonly known as the "good" fats, largely for their anti-inflammatory properties, which have been shown to protect against cardiovascular disease, neurodegenerative illnesses, arthritis, and autoimmune diseases, and may even act to enhance childhood learning.[31] They are considered essential fatty acids because the human body cannot make them. They must be obtained from the diet.

Two of the three types of dietary omega-3 fatty acids are docosahexaenoic acid (DHA) and eicosapentaenoic acid (EPA), both long-chain omega-3 fats. These fatty acids are made from a third type of short-chain omega-3 fatty acid known as alpha-linolenic acid (ALA), which serves as a building block for DHA and EPA.

Current recommendations by most experts and organizations urge the general public to eat more fish or take fish oil capsules to obtain adequate amounts of omega-3. While this typically provides sufficient omega-3 fatty acid intake, it also comes with the risk of ingesting toxic chemicals (dioxins, PCB's, chlorinated pesticides, and others) and high levels of mercury.[32] These pollutants have the potential to lead to negative effects on the nervous system, immune system, and even cardiovascular system.

A much safer way to obtain omega-3 fatty acids is directly from their source—plants. This is where fish obtain omega-3 fatty acids. Fish ingest algae or phytoplankton (rich in omega-3) from their natural sea environment. We in turn get omega-3 from eating fish. So why not cut out the middleman?

Plenty of healthy sources of omega-3 can be found in whole, plant-based foods such as chia seeds, hemps seeds, walnuts, or dark leafy greens. One to two tablespoons of seeds or a small handful of walnuts each day is sufficient in providing enough omega-3 to prevent a deficiency. This is equivalent to approximately 2 grams of omega-3.

Some people prefer to take omega-3 supplements. As I mentioned before, these supplements have their downsides. Flaxseed oil supplements should actually be avoided altogether (even though they're plant-based). They increase the risk of prostate cancer in men.[33] Flaxseed oil supplements are also devoid of fiber, lignans, and other health-promoting phytochemicals found in the original flaxseed. These health-promoting phytonutrients are removed during processing when the oil is extracted from the seed and put into pill form.

In contrast, ground flaxseed contains these beneficial substances and is one of the best sources of omega-3 you can consume. It has been associated with a reduction in both prostate and breast cancer.[34,35] This has been attributed to the rich source of dietary lignans found in flaxseeds.[36] Ground flaxseeds also provide a healthy dose of fiber, increasing bowel movements by up to 30 percent in some people.[37]

Another important study demonstrating the false sense of protection people believe they're getting from taking omega-3 supplements comes from a 2012 systemic review and meta-analysis published in the *Journal of the American Medical Association*. This review reported on the results of twenty randomized clinical trials. It included a total of 68,680 patients taking omega-3 supplementation and their risk of major cardiovascular events.[38] The review concluded, "Overall, omega-3 PUFA supplementation was not associated with a lower risk of all-cause mortality, cardiac death, sudden death, myocardial infarction, or stroke based on relative and absolute measures of association."

The important lesson learned in all of this is eating a diet rich in plant-based, whole foods is your best way to go. It should serve as your primary approach to achieving an optimal state of health. You should not be relying on the supplement industry to "sell" you on the fact that omega-3 pills are beneficial for you. In the end, nature knows best.

Supplements Worth Considering after Careful Review

Contrary to what you may be thinking, I am not against all supplements. I am actually an advocate for a few supplements, *but only if they're absolutely necessary* to avoid deficiencies leading to detrimental health consequences.

The Low Down on Vitamin D

Vitamin D has been heavily promoted in recent years for its wide array of health benefits. Studies have shown that optimal vitamin D levels are linked to a reduced incidence of many types of cancer, cardiovascular disease, diabetes, bacterial and viral infections, autoimmune diseases, osteoporosis, falls and fractures, dementia, congestive heart failure, and even adverse pregnancy outcomes.[39]

Vitamin D is thought to exert these additional health benefits—beyond its role of regulating calcium metabolism providing for strong, healthy bones—by acting as a hormone, thus regulating how various genes express themselves in the human body.[40]

In theory, avoiding a vitamin D deficiency would positively affect processes such as cellular growth, cardiovascular health, immune system activity, and other metabolic processes in the body, but the question remains: is this really the case? Are the litany of chronic diseases seen today an actual result of vitamin D deficiency *or* is vitamin D deficiency simply a consequence of these chronic diseases? More importantly, does supplementing with vitamin D produce any positive outcomes or is it merely a waste of time and money?

To answer these questions, the results of a few notable studies provided supply us with the best available evidence to date on vitamin D status, supplementing with vitamin D, and overall health. Much more debate is sure to come as the results of three major, randomized controlled trials are due out in the following years—VITAL (2017), FIND (2020), and VIDAL (2020).

Does vitamin D supplementation improve nonskeletal diseases such as diabetes, autoimmune disorders, cardiovascular disease, and others? It appears the answer so far is no. An article published in *The Lancet Diabetes & Endocrinology* December 2013 indicates that while low blood levels of vitamin D have been observed in a number of chronic illnesses, supplementing with vitamin D produced no risk reduction in these same diseases, even when individuals had a vitamin D deficiency before beginning supplementation.[41]

The one exception to this rule was in elderly patients (mainly women) who were diagnosed with a vitamin D deficiency at the beginning. These patients supplemented with vitamin D at 800 IU per day and slightly reduced their overall mortality rates. This echoes the results of a previous study indicating higher all-cause mortality rates in older individuals (greater than sixty-five) who had lower vitamin D levels.[42]

Another large-scale, meta-analysis published in the journal *PLoS ONE* December 2013 looked at vitamin D supplementation and overall mortality.[43] A total of forty-two randomized controlled trials with 85,466 patients were analyzed. The authors concluded vitamin D supplementation did have a beneficial effect on reducing overall mortality but only under the following conditions:

- Individuals with a vitamin D deficiency [25-(OH)D level < 20 ng/ml] at baseline (The Institute of Medicine currently sets the national guidelines for vitamin D status for the U.S. population. They state a vitamin D level greater than 20 ng/ml will cover the requirements of 97.5 percent of the population. Anything less than 20 ng/ml is considered a deficiency.)[44]
- In those supplementing with vitamin D at 800 IU per day or less for a minimum of three years or longer
- In elderly female patients younger than eighty years of age
- In those using cholecalciferol (vitamin D3) as opposed to ergocalciferol (vitamin D2)

The study went on to conclude that not enough data had yet been accumulated to determine the effects of vitamin D supplementation on mortality risk in males or young healthy adults.

Obviously, there is still much to be answered on the topic of vitamin D supplementation. As with any supplement you want to maximize your health while minimizing any adverse effects if supplementing. For now, it appears that unless you are elderly, and most likely female, with a vitamin D deficiency already diagnosed, then supplementation with vitamin D is of no benefit.

Vitamin B12—Don't Go Plant-Based Without It

Vitamin B12 is an essential vitamin requiring supplementation when following a whole foods, plant-based lifestyle. It's generally not present in most plant foods—other than a few processed breakfast cereals, which have been vitamin B12 fortified. These cereals are not the best choice when obtaining vitamin B12, though, as many of them consist of mostly refined grains and have a significant amount of sugar and salt added.

Other dietary sources of vitamin B12 include animal-based foods such as fish, poultry, beef, dairy, and eggs. These are also not the best choices for obtaining vitamin B12, as they've been found to contribute to a host of health problems as pointed out in chapter 10. This leaves supplementing in order to get enough B12 to avoid a deficiency.

Vitamin B12 fulfills three main functions in the human body. These include proper red blood cell formation, sound neurological functioning, and formation of our DNA.[45]

Deficiencies can lead to megaloblastic anemia, which is a red blood cell disorder.[46] This results in enlarged red blood cells and reduces their capacity to transport oxygen to tissues and organs throughout the body, which in turn results in severe fatigue and weakness. Neurological disorders, such as peripheral neuropathy, loss of coordination, psychiatric disorders, and even dementia, can also develop with a vitamin B12 deficiency.[47]

Many of these health conditions do not show up immediately, but after a period of approximately three to six years of inadequate vitamin B12 intake. It is at this time the body has used up its own stores of B12.[48] The key to avoiding a vitamin B12 deficiency is to replenish these stores on a daily basis.

Current guidelines from the Institute of Medicine (IOM) call for a Recommended Dietary Allowance of 2.4 mcg per day of vitamin B12 in healthy adults. This recommendation is far too low to properly restore ongoing B12 stores in the body. This was pointed out in a 2010 study in the *American Journal of Clinical Nutrition (AJCN)*.[49] The IOM based their recommendations on a small study, of only seven patients, conducted over six decades ago and found 2.4 mcg per day to be the minimum amount needed to prevent the occurrence of pernicious anemia—a disease of severe B12 deficiency. The IOM did not take into account, however, other health conditions that may occur from supplementing with such a small dose of B12. Based on the *AJCN* study, and a number of other large-scale studies, researchers determined a dose of between 4 and 10 mcg per day to be sufficient in maintaining normal B12 status in the general population.

Several different forms of vitamin B12 are available, including an intramuscular injection, topical patch, oral tablets, or sublingual tablets. Most individuals choose either an oral or sublingual (under the tongue) tablet. Please note only 1 to 2 percent of an oral dose of vitamin B12 is actually absorbed.[50] As a result, a higher dose is needed to obtain the 4 to 10 mcg/day recommended to prevent any possible deficiency. A dose of 1,000 mcg/day, or more, is usually sufficient in accomplishing this.[51]

Another consideration when choosing a B12 supplement is the form of the supplement. The most common form of vitamin B12 is cyanocobalamin, a synthetic version of this vitamin. Cyanocobalamin is broken down into two active forms of vitamin B12—methylcobalamin and 5-deoxyadenosylcobalamin. Your body uses both forms to maintain optimal health. Methylcobalamin is also available as a separate formulation but has no advantage over cyanocobalamin in healthy individuals. In those with chronic kidney disease methylcobalamin may be preferred over cyanocobalamin due to the prevention of potential toxic buildup of the metabolite cyanide, a byproduct of cyanocobalamin metabolism.[52]

Summing It All Up

The best way to recap supplementing is to take a closer look at the article from *Time* magazine by John Cloud, referenced in the introductory paragraph of this chapter. Cloud's goal was to find out whether or not supplementing is really worth it, evident by the title of his article—*Nutrition in a Pill?*

Conducting his own experiment, Cloud ordered a customized array of vitamins, minerals, and other nutraceutical products based on a state-of-the-art individualized assessment of his body's "needs" according to the supplement company he was ordering from. He received boxes full of supplements containing vitamins A, B6, B12, C, D3, E, K, and a host of other ingredients. For good measure, before starting this regimen, Cloud had his regular physician run baseline blood work for comparison. Throughout the course of his experiment he ended up taking a total of 3,300 pills (22 pills a day), over a five-month period, at a total cost of $1,200. So what happened after all of this?

Two things happened. First, only two of the thirty-one measurements from his blood work changed. His vitamin D level increased by 75 percent, due to the vitamin D supplement, and his HDL or "good choles-terol" increased by 46 percent. According to two separate physicians who reviewed Cloud's blood work, the rise in his HDL may or may not have been due to the supplements he was taking. Also, when asked about it, the company that supplied the supplements couldn't attribute the rise in HDL to their products.

The second thing that happened was Cloud experienced a weight gain of 10 pounds during his experiment. He readily admits after starting a powerful regimen of nutraceuticals he felt he was given a "license" to eat whatever he wanted. After all, he was getting everything he needed in a pill, right? It took Cloud three months to lose the added weight and get back on track eating right again. He subsequently summed up his experience with this quote, "You can take vitamins on the faith that they will make you better—and if you have a real vitamin deficiency, they will. But there's more science behind another way of getting your vitamins: eating right."

I've said it before and I'll say it again: human beings will never be able to outsmart Mother Nature when it comes to providing for your health. Fresh air, clean water, nutrient-rich plant-based foods, regular physical activity, quality sleep, and loving relationships are all that is required to achieve and maintain an optimal state of health. Pills, regardless of whether they're prescription drugs or the latest and greatest super vitamin, are medications at best and toxins at worst.

You might be wondering why a pharmacist would write a book that could effectively put himself out of business should people follow his advice. I'll tell you why. I wrote this book because I have a deep sense of love and compassion for my fellow human beings. My purpose in life is to do the

> **My purpose in life is to do the greatest amount of good for the most amount of people.**

greatest amount of good for the most amount of people. I've chosen to do this by entering the field of healthcare, helping others achieve the best health they can get.

I didn't know at the age of eighteen that becoming a pharmacist would fall far short of fulfilling these goals. This is exactly why I'm writing this book. I can't fix your medical problems. But I can care enough to share with you the knowledge I've accumulated up to this point in my life to help you fix them yourself. You've seen how this approach completely transforms people's lives. Now it's up to you to do something with it. I wish you the very best! May you live a long, happy, and healthy life!

Part III

Delicious Eats and Cool Treats

17

Healthy Plant-Based Recipes

"When baking, follow directions. When cooking,
go by your own taste."

—LAIKO BAHRS

Y
ou've now uncovered the missing link to longevity and excellent health. Now it's up to you to make it happen. Implementing a whole foods, plant-based lifestyle can be challenging if you don't know where to start. To help you, I've dedicated this chapter to sharing some of my favorite plant-based recipes.

These recipes contain little or no added salt, sugar, or fat. Some recipes do contain nuts and seeds, which are high-fat plant foods. As pointed out in chapter 9, these foods are rich in calories and may hinder some people's weight loss efforts. For these individuals it may be best to avoid these recipes or use them as occasional treats only.

The recipes that follow may take some time for your taste buds to adapt to. Generally, most people find this happens within three to four weeks. The key is to find recipes you enjoy. By doing so, you'll be more likely to stick with this lifestyle over the long term.

Time to dig in now! Don't forget to check out some of my favorite recipe websites at the end of this chapter for additional whole food, plant-based recipes.

Breakfast

Apple Cinnamon Oatmeal

Prep time: 2 minutes   Cook time: 6-7 minutes
Servings: 1

½   cup old-fashioned oats
1   cup water
⅓   cup raisins
3   slices of apple, chopped
⅓   cup chopped walnuts (optional)
1   teaspoon cinnamon
    Dash of nutmeg (optional)

Directions:
     Place oats, water, raisins, and chopped apple slices in small pot. Heat on stovetop on medium high for approximately 6-7 minutes or until semi-thick consistency achieved. Pour into bowl and top off with walnuts, cinnamon, and nutmeg.

Blueberry Banana Pancakes

Prep time: 5 minutes   Cook time: 2 minutes
Servings: 4

2   cups whole wheat flour
1   teaspoon baking soda
1   teaspoon baking powder
2   cups almond or soy milk
2   tablespoons unsweetened applesauce
1   banana, cut into small pieces
⅓   cup frozen blueberries

Directions:

Add flour, baking soda, and baking powder together in large bowl. Sift ingredients until well mixed. Add almond milk and applesauce to bowl. Mix until smooth consistency forms. Add in banana pieces and blueberries and stir well. You should have a smooth batter at this point.

Drop 2 heaping tablespoons onto a nonstick cooking pan or griddle on medium heat and flip when batter starts to bubble. Cook opposite side for approximately a minute and remove. Place finished pancakes in oven at 200 degrees to keep warm while cooking remaining pancakes. Pancakes should be fluffy and delicious. Serve with 100 percent pure maple syrup.

Ultimate Tofu Scramble

Prep time: 20 minutes   Cook time: 8 minutes
Servings: 3-4

1	14-ounce package extra-firm tofu
½	onion, chopped
½	bell pepper (any color), chopped
1	plum tomato, chopped
½	zucchini, chopped
4	ounces mushrooms, sliced
¼	teaspoon turmeric
1	teaspoon low-sodium soy sauce
¼	teaspoon cayenne pepper or black pepper

Directions:

Cut tofu into 8 pieces. Take one piece at a time and gently squeeze it between your hands to extract out extra moisture. About half the moisture should be removed now. Crumble tofu up with fingers and place in bowl. Repeat process with remaining tofu pieces.

Sauté onion, bell pepper, and mushrooms in large skillet with a tablespoon of water for approximately 5 minutes. Stir in turmeric and soy sauce and cook for approximately 30 seconds. Add tofu, tomatoes, zucchini, and pepper and stir-cook for 2-3 minutes. Serve immediately. Season with your favorite no-salt seasoning if preferred.

French Toast Topped With Mixed Berries

Prep time: 5 minutes   Cook time: 10-15 minutes
Servings: 8

1   ripe banana
1   cup almond milk
1   teaspoon apple pie spice (may substitute cinnamon)
8   slices whole grain bread

Directions:

Place banana, almond milk, and apple pie spice in blender and blend until completely liquefied. Pour mixture into a square dish. This is your batter.

Dip each slice of bread into the batter making sure to cover both sides. Immediately place bread onto nonstick skillet or grill and cook on medium heat for a few minutes before flipping. You'll want bread to be lightly browned on both sides. Placed finished French toast in oven at 200 degrees to keep warm while cooking remaining slices.

Top with a combination of your favorite berries (fresh or thawed frozen berries) along with 100 percent pure maple syrup.

Morning Almond Muesli Crunch

Prep time: 5 minutes
Servings: 1

1   cup old-fashioned oats
¼   cup sliced almonds
6   dates, pitted and chopped
1   tablespoon chia seeds
1   small peach, chopped
1   cup almond milk

Directions:

Place all ingredients into a bowl and mix well. Let sit overnight in the refrigerator to allow the oats to soak up the almond milk. Serve chilled.

Homestyle Hash Brown Casserole

Prep time: 30 minutes   Cook time: 30 minutes
Servings: 5-6

4	cups potatoes (prebaked), cubed
1	red onion, diced
2	cloves garlic, minced
1	bell pepper (any color), chopped
1	plum tomato, diced
1	cup mushrooms, chopped
1	cup spinach, finely chopped
3	tablespoons low-sodium vegetable stock
½	teaspoon black pepper
2	tablespoons dried basil
2	tablespoons parsley flakes
1	tablespoon paprika

Directions:

Preheat oven to 325 degrees. Sauté onions and garlic in 1 tablespoon of vegetable stock for approximately 5 minutes or until soft.

Lightly spray 9x13 baking dish with nonstick cooking spray. Add all ingredients together including onion and garlic in baking dish. Mix well and bake for 30 minutes. Let stand 5 minutes to cool before serving.

Smoothies and Shakes

Strawberry Mango Smoothie

1	cup frozen mango cubes
8	frozen strawberries
1	tablespoon ground flaxseed
1	cup almond or soy milk

Directions:

Blend all ingredients in high-powered blender until smooth.

Mean Green Smoothie

Recipe by Danah Veitenthal - www.pamperchef.biz/danahskitchen

½   apple
½   banana
5   strawberries
1   handful spinach
¼   cup water

Directions:
Blend all ingredients until smooth. For added sweetness add 1-2 pitted dates.

Chocolate Coconut Smoothie

1   frozen banana
1   handful kale
5   frozen strawberries
2   Medjool dates, pitted
2   tablespoons cocoa powder (may substitute with cacao powder)
2   tablespoons shredded unsweetened coconut
1   tablespoon cacao nibs (optional)
1   cup almond milk

Directions:
Blend all ingredients in high-powered blender until smooth.

Purple Power Shake

⅓ cup cranberries
1 handful kale
3 Medjool dates, pitted
¾ cup frozen mango cubes
1 cup frozen blueberries
1 cup pomegranate juice
   Splash of almond milk

Directions:
Blend all ingredients in high-powered blender until semi-thick consistency reached.

Blackberry Kiwi Smoothie

¼ whole pineapple, cubed and frozen
1 cup frozen blackberries
1 kiwi, peeled
1 pear
1 handful spinach
1 cup almond milk

Directions:
Blend all ingredients in high-powered blender until smooth.

Soups, Salads, Chili, & Stew

Danah's Ultimate Veggie Salad

Recipe by Danah Veitenthal - www.pamperchef.biz/danahskitchen

Prep time: 10-12 minutes
Servings: 2-3

	Kale, chopped (with stems removed)
	Bok Choy, diced (just the whites)
1	jicama, diced
½	ear of corn kernels (raw)
1	handful asparagus, diced
1	tomato, diced
½	avocado, sliced
2	carrots, julienne
1	cucumber, diced
1	bell pepper (any color), diced
1-2	tablespoons hemp seeds
1	small handful sunflower seeds
1	small handful pumpkin seeds
1-2	tablespoons nutritional yeast

Directions:
Toss all ingredients into a large bowl and mix well. Top salad off with Danah's Lemon Tahini Dressing (see Dressings, Dips, & Sauces) and toss salad again so that dressing and salad mixes together well. Serve and enjoy!

The Immune Booster Salad

Prep time: 6-7 minutes
Servings: 1-2

2	cups Arugula
2	cups Spring mix

1   cup shredded cabbage (any color)
1   carrot, sliced
1   plum tomato, diced
¾   cup broccoli, finely chopped
¾   cup cauliflower, finely chopped
½   cup red onion, chopped
⅛   cup sunflower seeds
½   avocado, sliced

Directions:

Toss all ingredients except for avocado into large salad bowl and mix well. Top with avocado slices. You can squeeze a fresh lemon or lime over top of salad to give it some zip if you wish. Also, try out a favorite dressing such as my Herbed Balsamic Tahini dressing.

Lentil Toss Salad

Prep time: 10 minutes   Cook time: 25 minutes
Servings: 8

1   cup uncooked lentils
2   cups water
2   cups cauliflower florets
2   cups broccoli florets
2   cups cucumbers, sliced and quartered
1   large carrot, grated
½   cup red onion, chopped
2   cups mushrooms, sliced
½   cup olives, sliced

Directions:

Place lentils and water in a large saucepan. Bring to a boil. Cover, reduce heat, and simmer 20 minutes or until lentils are tender. Drain well, and set aside to cool for a few minutes. In a serving bowl, toss lentils in with remaining ingredients. Serve and enjoy!

Omega-3-licious Fruit Salad

Prep time: 15-20 minutes
Servings: 4-5

1	apple, chopped
1	cup strawberries, chopped
1	orange, chopped
¼	cup blueberries
½	cup raisins
½	cup walnuts, chopped
½	cup unsweetened shredded coconut

Dressing:

3	tablespoons date syrup (may substitute agave)
1	tablespoon chia seeds
	Juice from 1 lime

Directions:
Add all fruit salad ingredients into a bowl and mix well. In a separate bowl, add date syrup, lime juice, and chia seeds. Whisk dressing together and pour over fruit salad. Mix well and serve.

Black-Eyed Pea Vegetable Gumbo Soup

Prep time: 5 minutes   Cook time: 10-15 minutes
Servings: 8

2	14.5-ounce cans no-salt-added diced tomatoes
2	15-ounce cans no-salt-added black-eyed peas
1	16-ounce package frozen vegetable gumbo mix
5	ounces frozen chopped onions
1	16-ounce package frozen turnip greens
1	16-ounce container low-sodium vegetable stock
1	small piece fresh ginger, peeled and finely chopped
1	teaspoon cayenne pepper
1	teaspoon garlic powder

2	teaspoons no-salt seasoning
½	teaspoon thyme

Directions:

Add all ingredients into a large pot. If you need to add more vegetable stock or water to cover the top of all the ingredients then do so as needed. Heat on high for approximately 10-15 minutes. Stir occasionally. Let soup cool for 5 minutes before serving.

Spicy Garden Chili

Prep time: 35 minutes   Cook time: 70 minutes
Servings: 10

4	stalks celery, chopped
1	large onion, chopped
1	green pepper, chopped
2	cloves fresh garlic, minced
1	14.5-ounce can low-sodium stewed tomatoes
1	15-ounce can no-salt-added tomato sauce
1	6-ounce can tomato paste
1	tablespoon Italian seasoning
1	tablespoon chili powder
1	teaspoon no-salt seasoning
½	teaspoon pepper
1	package low-sodium chili seasoning
2	15-ounce cans no-salt-added pinto beans
2	15-ounce cans no-salt-added red beans

Directions:

Add all chopped veggies into a large pot along with 1 tablespoon of water or vegetable broth and simmer for approximately 5 minutes. Add in remaining ingredients except beans and simmer for 1 hour, stirring occasionally. Add beans and simmer for 5-10 additional minutes. Warm to desired temperature and serve.

Butterbean Sweet Potato Stew (Crockpot Style)

Prep time: 30 minutes   Cook time: 6 hours
Servings: 6

1	15-ounce can low-sodium butterbeans, drained
2	garlic cloves, minced
1	fresh jalapeño, seeded and finely chopped
4	stalks celery, chopped
½	yellow pepper, chopped
½	red pepper, chopped
½	cup carrots, chopped
3	medium sweet potatoes, peeled and cubed
3	tablespoons tomato paste
¼	cup fresh parsley, finely chopped
4	cups low-sodium vegetable stock
½	teaspoon thyme
½	teaspoon cumin
½	teaspoon fennel
1	teaspoon dried basil
1	teaspoon paprika
1	teaspoon coriander
½	teaspoon black pepper

Directions:

Roast garlic in small amount of vegetable stock and then add to Crockpot. Place all other ingredients except the beans into the Crockpot. Cover and cook on low for 6 hours. Add beans to the Crockpot and cook for additional 30 minutes. Allow stew to cool for a few minutes before serving.

Black Bean Soup

Prep time: 20 minutes   Cook time: 40 minutes
Servings: 6-8

3	15-ounce cans no-salt-added black beans
3	cans water

2   tablespoons sherry (cooking wine)
2   cloves garlic, minced
1   yellow onion, chopped
1   Roma tomato, chopped
2   cups frozen okra, cut
2   cups kale, chopped
4   red potatoes (prebaked), cubed
½   teaspoon black pepper
1   tablespoon cumin
2   teaspoons oregano
1   teaspoon chili powder
1   teaspoon red pepper flakes
    Fresh basil to taste, chopped

Directions:

Note: Potatoes should be prebaked for this recipe and cut into small cubes. If you don't have time to prebake potatoes you can microwave them for 5 minutes.

Sauté garlic and onions in sherry (may substitute water) for 2-3 minutes in large pot. Add black pepper, cumin, and oregano. Continue to sauté for 2-3 more minutes or until onions are tender.

In a food processor or blender, blend one can of black beans and one can of water to form puree, add to the pot. Combine all other ingredients except kale. Bring to a boil. Reduce heat to medium low, cover, and cook for additional 30 minutes. Stir occasionally. Add kale, turn off heat, and let sit for additional 5 minutes before serving.

Split Pea and Root Vegetable Soup

Prep time: 30 minutes   Cook time: 45-60 minutes
Servings: 8-10

1   14-ounce package split peas
1   medium yucca root, cut into small cubes
1   large yellow onion, chopped
3   cloves garlic, minced
4   carrots, peeled and chopped
1   large leek, chopped (white and light green parts)

5	tomatillos, cut into quarter moons
2	tomatoes, chopped
1	jalapeño, finely chopped
1	bunch of cilantro, finely chopped
6	cups water
1	teaspoon celery seed
2	teaspoons no-salt seasoning
	Black pepper to taste

Directions:

In a large pot combine split peas and 3 cups of water. Heat on high for 10-15 minutes. While split peas are cooking prepare the rest of the vegetables. Add remaining ingredients to the pot. Lower heat to medium high and cook for additional 30-45 minutes. When yucca root and split peas are soft and tender the soup is done. Allow to cool for a few minutes before serving.

Burgers, Wraps, & Rolls

Black Bean & Brown Rice Burgers

Prep time: 15 minutes   Cook time: 10 minutes
Servings: 4

1	15-ounce can no-salt-added black beans, drained
1	cup cooked brown rice
1	small onion, diced
2	slices whole grain bread, crumbled (crust removed)
1	teaspoon garlic powder
1	teaspoon onion powder
½	teaspoon no-salt seasoning
½	teaspoon pepper
½	teaspoon red pepper flakes (optional)
	Whole grain or whole wheat buns or pita pockets

Directions:

Sauté onions in a cooking pan until soft. While waiting for onions to tenderize, mash beans in a large bowl until almost smooth. Add onions, bread crumbles, and all seasonings together with the beans and mix. Add small portions of cooked brown rice to form a thick consistent mixture. This is your patty mix.

Form bean and brown rice mixture into patties approximately one-half inch thick. Fry patties in a nonstick skillet. Serve with 100 percent whole grain buns or pita pockets. Top with lettuce leaf, tomato, mustard, Worcestershire (no anchovy) sauce, or other toppings of choice.

Grilled Portobello Mushroom Burger with Caramelized Onions

Prep time: 10 minutes   Cook time: 10 minutes
Servings: 2

2   portobello mushrooms (stems removed)
1   sweet onion, sliced
1   Roma tomato, sliced
2   romaine lettuce leaves
1   avocado, sliced
2   whole grain hamburger buns or 4 slices whole grain bread
2   tablespoons low-sodium vegetable broth
2   tablespoons low-sodium soy sauce

Directions:

In a bowl, add together veggie broth and soy sauce. Brush mushrooms with sauce. Place mushrooms in a nonstick skillet and grill over medium heat. Cook until tender, about 8-10 minutes, turning once. You may need to add a small amount of sauce to coat pan if necessary.

While mushrooms are cooking, in a separate pan add onion slices topped with remainder of sauce mix. Cook on medium heat until onions are golden brown, about 8 minutes.

Place mushrooms on top of bun. Top with onions, sliced tomato, avocado slices, and lettuce. Serve with your favorite condiments.

Whole Grain DLT Sandwich

Prep time: 5 minutes
Servings: 1

2	slices whole grain sprouted bread
2	tablespoons hummus
1	Roma tomato, sliced
1	large leaf romaine lettuce
½	cup dulse (sea vegetable)

Directions:

Spread hummus onto both pieces of whole grain bread. Layer sliced tomato, lettuce, and dulse between bread.

If you prefer crispy dulse in your sandwich then place dulse in oven for approximately 5 minutes at 250 degrees before adding to sandwich.

Black Bean Quinoa Wraps

Prep time: 15 minutes   Cook time: 20 minutes
Servings: 6-8

1	package of whole wheat wraps (6-8 wraps)
1	cup Inca red quinoa
2½	cups water
1	15-ounce can no-salt-added black beans, drained
5	scallions, finely chopped
1	clove garlic, minced
3	ounces sun dried tomatoes, chopped
1	teaspoon chili powder
2	teaspoon no-salt seasoning
1	teaspoon onion powder

Directions:

Cook quinoa according to package instructions using 2 cups of water. While quinoa is cooking prep scallions, garlic, and sun dried tomatoes.

Once quinoa has absorbed all moisture, add one-half cup water, beans, scallions, garlic, sun dried tomatoes, and seasonings. Stir well. Heat on medium low for approximately 5 minutes.

Warm whole wheat wraps in oven for 1-2 minutes at 170 degrees. Spread 1-2 tablespoons of Cashew Sour Cream (see Dressings, Dips, & Sauces) onto wrap. Next, add desired amount of black bean quinoa mixture and roll wrap up. Serve and enjoy!

Portobello Fajita Wraps

Recipe by Holly Yzquierdo - http://myplantbasedfamily.com

Prep time: 30 minutes   Cook time: 10 minutes

	Whole wheat tortillas
1	portobello mushroom
½	onion, sliced
1	bell pepper, sliced
1	cup low-sodium vegetable broth
1	teaspoon garlic powder
1	teaspoon onion powder
1	teaspoon chili powder
1	teaspoon Worcestershire sauce
1	teaspoon liquid smoke
1	tablespoon balsamic vinegar

Directions:

Remove the stem and slice mushrooms. If you are making Portobello steaks, you don't need to slice mushrooms, just remove the stem. Mix the remaining ingredients together and allow mushroom and veggie slices to soak for approximately 30 minutes. Broil the mushroom slices for 5 minutes, then flip and broil for 5 additional minutes. Remove from oven and allow to cool slightly.

These are great served in a warm tortilla. They're even better with fresh guacamole and salsa. You can also top a salad with these, and even add roasted corn.

Raw Taco Wrap

Recipe by Rebecca Joy

Prep time: 15 minutes
Servings: 5

5	large collard leaves
1	bunch cilantro, chopped
1	jalapeño, diced
1	avocado, sliced
1	large tomato, chopped
1	onion, chopped
1	lemon

Taco "meat"

2	cups walnuts
⅔	cup kalamata olives
2½	tablespoons chili powder
1	teaspoon annatto spice
1½	teaspoons cumin
½	teaspoon marjoram leaves
1	teaspoon paprika
¼	teaspoon cayenne
½	teaspoon garlic powder

Directions:

To make taco "meat," add walnuts, olives, and spices into a food processor. Process until gritty texture achieved. Spread 2-3 spoonfuls onto collard leaf. Add remaining veggies on top of "meat" just as if you were to make a regular taco. Freshly squeeze some lemon juice onto veggies and roll collard leaf up to make wrap.

You may also substitute your favorite dressing or salsa in place of the freshly squeezed lemon if preferred.

Dressings, Dips, & Sauces

Danah's Lemon Tahini Dressing

Recipe by Danah Veitenthal - www.pamperchef.biz/danahskitchen

⅛   cup water
1   lemon, juiced
2   tablespoons tahini
¼   teaspoon salt

Directions:
Add all ingredients into a bowl and mix well. Serve over any salad or use with Danah's Ultimate Veggie Salad recipe.

Cashew Fig Infused Dressing

½   cup cashews
½   cup almond or soy milk
2   tablespoons fig infused vinegar
2   tablespoons mustard (flavor of choice)
1   tablespoon low-sodium tamari sauce
1   clove garlic, minced
1   tablespoon Mrs. Dash table blend seasoning
2   dates, pitted
⅓   cup water

Directions:
Place all ingredients in high-powered blender and blend until smooth.

Tahini Dill Salad Dressing

½   cup tahini
2   tablespoons mustard
1   tablespoon rice or balsamic vinegar
2   tablespoons low-sodium soy sauce

½ cup water
1 teaspoon dill weed

Directions:
Place all ingredients in a bowl and whisk until thoroughly mixed. If you want a creamier consistency then use less water.

Tangy Walnut Balsamic Dressing

½ cup balsamic vinegar
¼ cup walnuts
¼ cup mustard
1 tablespoon low-sodium tamari sauce
2 Medjool dates, pitted
Juice of 1 lemon

Directions:
Blend all ingredients in blender until mostly smooth. Don't blend too long otherwise dressing will become thick. You want a creamy, smooth consistency with this recipe.

Spicy Brown Mustard Dressing

¾ cup water
¼ cup spicy brown mustard
¼ cup tahini
1 tablespoon tamari
1 tablespoon lemon juice
1 teaspoon no-salt seasoning

Directions:
Add all ingredients into a blender or food processor and blend until smooth.

Herbed Balsamic Tahini Dressing

⅓ cup balsamic vinegar
½ cup tahini
1 cup water
1 clove garlic, minced
¼ cup fresh parsley
1 tablespoon dried basil
1 teaspoon ground oregano
½ teaspoon no-salt seasoning
½ teaspoon black pepper
2 teaspoons dijon mustard

Directions:
Add all ingredients into blender or food processor and blend until smooth.

Lemon Garlic Hummus

Prep time: 10 minutes

1 15-ounce can no-salt-added garbanzo beans, drained
2 cloves garlic, crushed
1 tablespoon lemon juice
1 tablespoon low-sodium soy sauce
1 tablespoon mustard
¼ cup tahini
Pinch of cayenne pepper

Directions:
Add all ingredients into blender or food processor and blend until smooth. If consistency is clumpy or thick then add a small amount of water to obtain a smoother consistency. Refrigerate any unused portion for up to three days.

Cashew Sour Cream

Prep time: 5 minutes

1 cup cashews
2 tablespoons lemon juice
1 tablespoon apple cider vinegar
⅓ cup water

Directions:
Add all ingredients into blender and blend until mixture reaches thick, creamy texture. Add more water if needed to reduce thickness. Use as substitute for sour cream. This recipe is perfect for putting on wraps or tacos.

Spicy Mango Salsa

Prep time: 15-20 minutes
Servings: 4

1 mango, peeled, pitted, and cubed
½ Florida avocado, peeled, pitted, and diced or 1 large Hass avocado
½ red onion, chopped
1 habañero pepper, seeded and finely diced
½ Roma tomato, diced
3 tablespoons fresh cilantro, chopped
½ lime

Directions:
Place all ingredients in medium size bowl. Squeeze lime over ingredients and mix well. You can add pepper to taste if desired, but this is one hot salsa dish already. For a tamer version try using only half of a habañero pepper.

Main Entrees

Collard Greens & Red Bell Pepper Tempeh

Prep time: 15 minutes   Cook time: 35 minutes
Servings: 2-3

8	ounces collard greens
1	8-ounce package tempeh, cut into bite size pieces
1	red bell pepper, chopped
1	shallot, chopped
3	cloves garlic, minced
½	cup shiitake mushrooms, chopped
½	cup fresh cilantro, chopped
1	tablespoon low-sodium tamari
1	tablespoon lemon juice
½	cup water
2	tablespoons low-sodium vegetable stock
½	teaspoon red pepper flakes
¼	teaspoon black pepper
½	teaspoon no-salt seasoning

Directions:

After rinsing collard greens place them in a large pot with enough water to submerge them. Cover and bring to boil. Lower heat and simmer for 10 minutes. Drain and set aside.

While collards are cooking, place tempeh, tamari, lemon juice, and water into a large skillet. Cover and bring to boil. Lower heat and simmer for 10 minutes. Drain any excess liquid.

While tempeh is cooking, place shallot, garlic, and vegetable stock in a small skillet. Sauté for 3-4 minutes and then add to tempeh (already drained) and mushrooms. Sauté tempeh, mushrooms, shallot, and garlic for 5 minutes, adding a little vegetable stock if needed to keep from drying out. Add in cooked collards, cilantro, red bell pepper, red pepper flakes, black pepper, and no-salt seasoning. Sauté on medium low for 10-12 minutes. Serve immediately.

Chickpea Vegetable Medley with Brown Rice

Recipe by Rebecca Joy

Prep time: 15 minutes   Cook time: 40 minutes
Servings: 4

1	zucchini, cut into quarter moons
1	red onion, chopped
1	bell pepper (any color), diced
1	15-ounce can no-salt-added garbanzo beans
1	14.5-ounce can no-salt-added diced tomatoes
1	15-ounce can no-salt-added tomato sauce
2	cloves garlic, minced
½	teaspoon oregano
1	teaspoon Mrs. Dash table blend seasoning
1	tablespoon low-sodium vegetable stock

Directions:

Cook 2 cups of brown rice according to package instructions and set aside. Sauté onions and garlic in pan with vegetable stock for 5 minutes or until onions are semi-soft. Add chopped veggies and sauté for additional 15 minutes. Add tomato sauce, diced tomatoes, and spices and cook for 10-15 minutes.

While vegetable medley above is cooking, heat chickpeas in a separate pot on medium heat until boiling. Reduce heat and simmer for 10 minutes and then drain.

Add brown rice, vegetable medley, and chickpeas in large bowl and mix. Serve immediately.

Veggie Pita Pizza

Prep time: 20-25 minutes   Cook time: 12 minutes
Servings: 6

6   whole wheat pita rounds (Ezekiel 4:9 pocket bread is a great choice)
2   cups homemade "cheese" sauce
8   ounces homemade pizza sauce
     Freshly chopped veggies (tomatoes, bell peppers, broccoli, zucchini, onions, olives, etc.)

Homemade pizza sauce
1   8-ounce can no-salt-added tomato sauce
1   tablespoon Italian seasoning
1   teaspoon onion powder
½   teaspoon garlic powder
1   teaspoon no-salt seasoning

Homemade "cheese" sauce
1   cup water
¼   cup tahini
¼   cup cashews
2   tablespoons nutritional yeast
½   teaspoon onion powder
¼   teaspoon garlic powder
1   tablespoon lemon juice
¼   cup cornstarch
1   teaspoon no-salt seasoning

Directions for "cheese" sauce:
    Blend all ingredients (except half-cup of water reserved for later) until smooth. Pour mixture into small pot and add remaining half-cup water. Heat until boiling. Reduce heat to low and simmer until sauce thickens, stirring regularly.

Directions for pizza:
    Preheat oven to 375 degrees. Place pita rounds on nonstick baking sheet. Spread enough homemade pizza sauce to cover pita. Spread 2 tablespoons "cheese" sauce on top of pizza sauce. Add preferred choice of chopped veggies on the pita rounds. Bake 12 minutes. Cool before serving.

Sweet & Sour Vegetable Stir-Fry

Prep time: 20 minutes   Cook time: 20 minutes
Servings: 4

1	zucchini, cut into half moons
1	yellow squash, cut into half moons
½	bell pepper (any color), chopped
2	cups broccoli
2	carrots, sliced
1	cup snap peas
1	medium onion, chopped
½	clove garlic, minced
1	small tomato, cut into wedges
1	cup pineapple chunks
1	8-ounce package tempeh, cut into cubes

Sweet & sour stir-fry sauce

1	cup pineapple juice
2	tablespoons rice vinegar or distilled white vinegar
1	tablespoon agave
¼	cup dry sherry
1¼	tablespoons cornstarch
2	tablespoons low-sodium soy sauce
¼	teaspoon ginger (optional)

Directions:

Place all ingredients for sweet & sour sauce into a bowl and whisk together.

Sauté onions and garlic in a wok with a small amount of sauce over medium low heat for approximately 5 minutes or until soft. Add remaining ingredients except tomatoes and pineapple, along with remainder of sauce. Cook over medium heat for 10-12 minutes, stirring frequently. Add tomato wedges and pineapple chunks and cook for an additional 5 minutes. Serve immediately.

Note: You may substitute firm or extra firm tofu or seitan for the tempeh if you prefer. You may also wish to serve stir-fry over a bed of brown rice or rice noodles.

Avocado Tacos

Prep time: 30 minutes   Cook time: 10 minutes
Servings: 12

12 Whole grain tortillas (Ezekiel 4:9 sprouted grain tortillas are good)
1   ripe avocado, peeled and seeded
1   medium onion, julienne
2   large green bell peppers, julienne
2   large red bell peppers, julienne
1   cup fresh cilantro, finely chopped
1   15-ounce can no-salt-added pinto beans
1½ cups fresh tomato salsa
1   cup no-salt-added diced tomatoes
⅓ cup onions, diced
1   clove garlic, minced
2   teaspoons cilantro
⅓ teaspoon jalapeño peppers, finely chopped
    Juice from 1 lime
    Pinch of cumin

Directions:

To prepare salsa, mix all ingredients in bowl and refrigerate in advance.

Heat pinto beans on medium low heat for 10 minutes and drain when finished. While beans are warming, lightly sauté onion and bell peppers in a skillet with small amount of water or vegetable broth. Cut avocado into 12 slices.

Warm tortillas in oven on low for approximate 5 minutes and then fill with peppers, onions, beans, cilantro, salsa, and avocado slices.

Bok Choy and Bell Pepper Quinoa

Prep time: 10-15 minutes   Cook time: 20-30 minutes
Servings: 4

1   cup quinoa, rinsed
2   cups water
2   tablespoons low-sodium vegetable broth

8 ounces mushrooms, sliced
1 yellow bell pepper, chopped
1 red bell pepper, chopped
5 leaves bok choy, chopped
½ inch piece ginger, minced
1 lime, zested and juiced
1 teaspoon no-salt seasoning
3 tablespoons low-sodium tamari or soy sauce
   Pepper to taste

Directions:

Add water and quinoa to pot, simmer for 20-30 minutes until fully cooked. Quinoa will appear fluffy when fully cooked. Do not stir while cooking.

While quinoa is cooking, add vegetable broth and mushrooms to a large pan and heat on medium until mushrooms are soft. Add peppers and cook approximately 5 minutes. Add bok choy, continue to cook until leaves start to wilt. Add ginger, lime zest, and no-salt seasoning and stir. Next, add cooked quinoa and gently stir through vegetables.

Combine lime juice and tamari sauce in bowl and mix together. Pour over quinoa and vegetable mixture, stir and add pepper to taste. Garnish with fresh parsley or cilantro before serving.

Pineapple Chickpea Curry

Prep time: 15 minutes   Cook time: 10 minutes
Servings: 2

1   bag precooked brown rice (Success brand)
1   shallot, diced
3   cloves garlic, minced
2   tablespoons low-sodium vegetable broth
½   red bell pepper, chopped
½   orange bell pepper, chopped
½   teaspoon ground turmeric
2½ teaspoons ground cumin
½   teaspoon cayenne pepper
½   teaspoon ground coriander
½   teaspoon black pepper

2	tablespoons low-sodium soy sauce
1	15-ounce can no-salt-added garbanzo beans
½	fresh pineapple, cubed
½	cup fresh cilantro, chopped
3	tablespoons lemon juice (freshly squeezed is best)
3	tablespoons coconut milk (optional)

Directions:

Cook rice according to package instructions. This should take approximately 10 minutes.

While rice is cooking, add vegetable broth, shallot, and garlic to frying pan. Sauté for 1 minute on medium high heat. Add red and orange pepper, soy sauce, all spices except black pepper, and 1 tablespoon water to frying pan and sauté for additional 2-3 minutes. Add garbanzo beans and mix well. Cook for approximately 5 minutes.

Add pineapple, lemon juice, black pepper, and cilantro. You may also add coconut milk at this time if using in recipe. Stir well and cook 1-2 additional minutes. Serve over brown rice. If more of a salty taste is preferred then pour small amount of soy sauce over final dish.

Easy Mexican Rice and Bean Casserole

Recipe by Holly Yzquierdo - http://myplantbasedfamily.com

Prep time: 5 minutes   Cook time: 50-90 minutes
Servings: 6-8

1	cup brown rice
2½	cups water (3 cups for casserole version)
1	8-ounce can of tomato sauce
1	teaspoon onion powder
1	teaspoon chili powder
½	teaspoon garlic powder
½	teaspoon cumin
2	cups cooked pinto or black beans (or 1 can drained beans)
1	cup corn (optional)

Directions For Casserole Version

Preheat oven to 350 degrees. Add all ingredients into a 9x15 casserole dish and stir gently. Bake for 60-90 minutes until rice is tender.

Directions For Stove Top Version

Add all ingredients except beans into a pan (I use a skillet) and cover, cooking over medium heat. Stir occasionally, adding more water if necessary. Rice should be nice and soft after 45 minutes, add the beans and corn if using, then stir to mix. Heat until everything is warm. Serve on a bed of greens with a bit of guacamole and homemade pico or salsa if desired.

Desserts

Chocolate Coconut Oat Bars

Prep time: 10-15 minutes   Cook time: 15-17 minutes
Servings: 15 bars

1   15-ounce can no-salt-added pinto beans
½   cup almond butter (may substitute peanut butter)
½   cup agave
¼   cup unsweetened applesauce
1   teaspoon vanilla extract
½   teaspoon nutmeg
1½   cups old-fashioned oats
½   cup whole wheat flour
½   cup cacao powder (may substitute cocoa powder)
1   cup unsweetened shredded coconut

Directions:

Combine beans, almond butter, agave, applesauce, vanilla, and nutmeg into food processor. Blend until smooth. Add oats, flour, and cacao powder. Pulse until all ingredients are well mixed. Add coconut and pulse until mixed well. If mixture is too dry then add a small amount of water to provide spreadable consistency. If mixture is too wet then add a small amount of flour.

Lightly spray a 9x13 pan with nonstick cooking spray. Spread mixture evenly in pan.

Bake at 350 degrees for 15-17 minutes. Let cool for 5-10 minutes before serving.

Pumpkin Cake/Cupcakes

Recipe by Holly Yzquierdo - http://myplantbasedfamily.com

Prep time: 5 minutes   Cook time: 20-40 minutes

2   cups whole wheat pastry flour
1   teaspoon baking powder
½   teaspoon baking soda
1   teaspoon pumpkin pie spice
1½   cups pumpkin (or 1 can)
1   cup maple syrup
1   teaspoon vanilla
½   cup almond milk
     Vegan chocolate chips (optional)

Directions:

Preheat oven to 350 degrees. In a large bowl mix the first 5 ingredients. In medium bowl mix the remaining ingredients, except chocolate chips if using. Pour wet ingredients into the dry ingredients and mix.

Grease 9-inch cake pan or use cupcake liners. Pour into pan and bake until done, 30-40 minutes for the 9-inch cake pan or 15-20 minutes for cupcakes.

Chocolate Banana Creme Pie

Prep time: 15 minutes
Servings: 8 slices

Crust:
¾   cup Medjool dates, pitted
1¾   cups walnuts

Pie filling:
3   frozen bananas
1   cup cashews
⅓   cup cacao powder
¼   cup almond butter
¾   cup almond milk

½   teaspoon vanilla extract

Directions:

To make crust put walnuts and dates into food processor and process until finely ground with a gritty texture. Pour mixture into pie pan and press evenly. Place the piecrust in freezer while making pie filling.

To make pie filling place all ingredients into high-powered blender. Blend until a thick, creamy consistency is reached. Pour filling into piecrust and spread evenly. Place pie in refrigerator and let chill for at least 15 minutes before serving.

Hemp Chia Nutty Bars

Recipe by Victoria Dool

Prep time: 10 minutes   Cook time: 40 minutes
Servings: 12 bars

1	cup walnuts
1	cup pecans
1	cup sunflower seeds, unsalted
1	cup hemp seeds
¼	cup chia seeds
2	ripe bananas
4	dates, pitted
2	teaspoons agave

Directions:

Preheat oven to 200 degrees. Lightly spray 9x13 pan with nonstick cooking spray.

Place walnuts, pecans, and sunflower seeds into food processor. Pulse until nuts are finely chopped. Pour nut mixture into a large bowl and set aside. Place bananas, dates, and agave into food processor and pulse until smooth and creamy. Pour banana mix over nut mixture set aside earlier. Add hemp and chia seeds, mix thoroughly.

Pour mixture into pan and spread evenly with spatula. Bake for 40 minutes. Cool for approximately 5 minutes before serving. Cut into rectangles to make bars. Eat the bars fresh or refrigerate for later.

Apple Berry Crisp

Prep time: 10 minutes   Cook time: 25 minutes
Servings: 4

1   apple, cored and chopped
1   cup frozen mixed berries (thawed)
½   cup raisins
6   dates, pitted and chopped
½   cup pecans or walnuts, finely chopped
⅔   cup old-fashioned oats
1   tablespoon pecan meal
½   teaspoon cinnamon
¼   teaspoon nutmeg
3   tablespoons applesauce
1   teaspoon freshly grated ginger
¼   cup water

Directions:
Preheat oven to 375 degrees. Lightly spray 2-quart rectangular baking dish with nonstick cooking spray. Add berries, apple chunks, and raisins.

In separate bowl combine dates, nuts, oats, pecan meal, cinnamon, nutmeg, applesauce, and ginger. Stir until mixed well. Pour mixture into baking dish, add water and mix thoroughly. Bake for 25 minutes. Let cool for approximately 5 minutes before serving.

Double Chocolate Brownies

Prep time: 20 minutes
Servings: 9 bars

1½   cups walnuts
½   cup unsweetened shredded coconut
2   cups Medjool dates, pitted
⅔   cup cacao powder

Frosting:
½ large avocado
⅓ cup fresh raspberries
1¼ ounces agave
⅛ cup cacao powder
1 teaspoon vanilla extract
¼ teaspoon cinnamon

Directions:

Add walnuts, coconut, and dates to food processor and process for approximately 15-20 seconds. Add cacao powder and process until a consistent gritty texture is formed. Pour mixture into a 2-quart baking dish and press until solid brownie base is formed.

Add avocado, raspberries, agave, cacao powder, vanilla, and cinnamon to food processor and process until thick, creamy frosting is formed. Spread frosting over the top of brownie base. Cut into squares and serve.

Peanut Butter Ice Cream

Prep time: 5 minutes

3 frozen bananas
¼ cup unsweetened cacao powder (or cocoa powder)
¼ cup natural peanut butter (or almond butter)
½ cup almond milk

Directions:

Place all ingredients into high-powered blender. Blend until thick, creamy consistency achieved. It should have the perfect texture of soft serve ice cream to it. Scoop into bowls or cups. Place in freezer for a few minutes to let chill before serving if desired.

Additional Whole Food, Plant-Based Recipe Websites

Straight Up Food - www.straightupfood.com

Fat Free Vegan - http://fatfreevegan.com

Happy Herbivore - http://happyherbivore.com

McDougall recipes - www.drmcdougall.com/newsletter/recipeindex.html

Healthy Girl's Kitchen - http://www.healthygirlskitchen.com

Plant-Powered Kitchen - http://plantpoweredkitchen.com

The Blissful Chef - http://theblissfulchef.com

Fuhrman recipes - http://www.drfuhrman.com/library/recipes.aspx

NutritionMD - www.nutritionmd.org

Unprocessed - www.eatunprocessed.com/dietitian.html

4Leaf Program - http://4leafprogram.com/recipes

Forks Over Knives - www.ForksOverKnives.com

The China Study - http://www.thechinastudy.com/category/recipe/

My Plant-Based Family - http://myplantbasedfamily.com

Resources

Books

The China Study - T. Colin Campbell, PhD, and Thomas M. Campbell II
Whole - T. Colin Campbell, PhD, and Howard Jacobson, PhD
The Low-Carb Fraud - T. Colin Campbell, PhD, and Howard Jacobson, PhD
The Starch Solution - John McDougall, MD
The McDougall Program - John McDougall, MD
The McDougall Program for Maximum Weight Loss - John McDougall, MD
Dr. McDougall's Digestive Tune Up - John McDougall, MD
Prevent and Reverse Heart Disease - Caldwell Esselstyn, Jr., MD
Vegan Nutrition - Michael Klaper, MD
Eat To Live - Joel Fuhrman, MD
Eat For Health - Joel Fuhrman, MD
Disease-Proof Your Child - Joel Fuhrman, MD
Super Immunity - Joel Fuhrman, MD
The End of Diabetes - Joel Fuhrman, MD
Dr. Neal Barnard's Program for Reversing Diabetes - Neal Barnard, MD
21-Day Weight Loss Kickstart - Neal Barnard, MD
Power Foods For The Brain - Neal Barnard, MD
Solving America's Healthcare Crisis - Pamela Popper, PhD, ND
Food Over Medicine - Pamela Popper, PhD, ND, and Glen Merzer
The Engine 2 Diet - Rip Esselstyn
My Beef With Meat - Rip Esselstyn
Healthy At 100 - John Robbins
The Food Revolution - John Robbins
Diet for a New America - John Robbins
The Spectrum - Dean Ornish, MD
The Perfect Formula Diet - Janice Stanger, PhD

Books *(continued)*

Unprocessed - Chef AJ
Whitewash - Joseph Keon
Fit Quickies - Lani Muelrath
Senior Fitness - Ruth Heidrich, PhD
A Race For Life - Ruth Heidrich, PhD
Lifelong Running - Ruth Heidrich, PhD
The Pleasure Trap - Douglas Lisle, PhD, and Alan Goldhamer, DC
Mad Cowboy - Howard Lyman with Glen Merzer
No More Bull! - Howard Lyman with Glen Merzer
Healthy Eating, Healthy World - J. Morris Hicks with J. Stanfield Hicks
Keep It Simple, Keep It Whole - Matthew Lederman, MD, and Alona Pulde, MD
The Complete Idiot's Guide to Plant-Based Nutrition - Julieanna Hever, MS, RD, CPT
Becoming Vegan: Express Edition - Brenda Davis, RD, and Vesanto Melina, RD
Becoming Vegan: Comprehensive Edition - Brenda Davis, RD, and Vesanto Melina, RD

DVDs

Forks Over Knives
Food, Inc.
Fat, Sick & Nearly Dead
Foodmatters
Vegucated
Supersize Me
To Your Health
King Corn
Processed People
Planeat
Fast Food Nation
The Beautiful Truth
Simply Raw
Jeff Novick's Fast Food Vol 1: The Basics
Jeff Novick's Fast Food Vol 2: Burgers & Fries
Jeff Novick's Fast Food Vol 3: Shopping School
Osteoporosis Protection For Life - Joel Fuhrman, MD
Dr. McDougall's Total Health Solution
Latest In Clinical Nutrition - Michael Greger, MD
Tackling Diabetes with Dr. Neal Barnard
Get Healthy Now! - Vegsource.com
Digestion Made Easy - Michael Klaper, MD

DVDs *(continued)*

Salt, Sugar, and Oil: The Good the Bad and the Ugly - Michael Klaper, MD

Understanding Your Blood Test Results - Michael Klaper, MD

Healing Clinics

www.drmcdougall.com - Health and Medical Center of John McDougall, MD

www.wellnessforum.com - Health and Wellness Clinic of Pam Popper, ND

www.healthpromoting.com - True North Health Center of Alan Goldhamer, DC

www.ornishspectrum.com - Medical Lifestyle Programs of Dean Ornish, MD

www.drfuhrman.com - Medical Associates Clinic of Joel Fuhrman, MD

www.chiphealth.com - Complete Health Improvement Program founded by Hans Diehl, PhD

www.hippocratesinst.org - Lifestyle Transformation Program directed by Brian Clement, PhD, and Anna Clement, PhD

Helpful Websites

www.plantbasedpharmacist.com

www.vegsource.com

www.dresselstyn.com

www.pcrm.org

www.doctorklaper.com

www.nealbarnard.org

www.forksoverknives.com

www.healthyeatinghealthyworld.com

www.pursueahealthyyou.com

www.nomeatathlete.com

www.farms2forks.com

www.happycow.net

www.johnrobbins.info

www.passthekale.com

www.lanimuelrath.com

www.happyhealthylonglife.com

www.thefoodpharmacy.com

www.wholevana.com

www.thedrdonshow.com

www.nakedfoodmagazine.com

www.stlveggirl.com

http://nutritionstudies.org

Helpful Websites *(continued)*

http://jeffnovick.com
http://nutritionfacts.org
http://engine2diet.com
http://perfectformuladiet.com
http://myplantbasedfamily.com
http://ruthheidrich.com
http://vegcoach.com
http://cancerdecisions.com
http://yummyplants.com
http://theplantrx.com
http://plantivores.com
http://plantbasedresearch.org

Acknowledgments

This book would not have happened without the love and support of my family. I want to thank my father, Terry Rudolph, and my mother, Jeanie Daughdrill, for their unwavering support and guidance along the way. I thank my two brothers, Blake and Taylor Rudolph, for all their words of encouragement as I dedicated countless hours to the completion of this project. Thank you, Blake, for providing your ideas on how to improve this book; they were influential in adding an entire chapter of material to the final product.

I also owe a special thank you to my personal physician and dear friend Dr. Salvatore DeLellis for planting a seed in me. If not for you, none of this would have been possible. Your introduction of lifestyle medicine and plant-based nutrition to me has changed my life forever. I no longer fear the chronic diseases that plague the lives of so many in this world. Instead, I know without a doubt that my future is one of optimal health as I put into practice what I have learned because of you. Your efforts have also changed the lives of hundreds and even thousands of others as I carry this information forward in hopes of providing them with the same life-changing message you gave me.

I have many close friends who have also been an unending source of inspiration in the writing of this book. I couldn't have gotten to where I am today without you. A special thank you to Rebecca Joy for providing daily motivation when I thought I couldn't go any further. To Amber Hoffman, I'm forever grateful for all your unselfishness with the time you dedicated in reading each and every chapter as it unfolded. I also thank my friend Janice Stanger for her expertise and counsel with this project. You took me under your wings and literally helped me fly with this first piece of literary work.

Many other friends and colleagues too numerous to name have made this project possible by inspiring me with their much-appreciated words of encouragement, suggestions, and tips. They include my lifelong college friends, my St. Louis and Florida compadres, and my fellow hospital coworkers. Thank you for all the support you've given me along the way.

About the Author

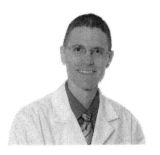

With over a decade of experience in the field of pharmacy, **Dustin Rudolph, PharmD,** is a clinical pharmacist currently practicing in an acute care hospital setting. He graduated with a Doctor of Pharmacy degree in 2002 from North Dakota State University in Fargo. His professional experience covers a multitude of patient populations including neonatal, pediatric, cardiac, orthopedic, oncology, diabetic, intensive care, and geriatric patients, just to name a few.

In 2009, Dr. Rudolph adopted a vegetarian diet, and then a whole foods, plant-based diet (vegan) a year later. He founded his website (www.PlantBasedPharmacist.com) with a goal of providing reliable, high-quality, evidence-based health and wellness information to improve the knowledge of both patients and medical professionals.

He continued his education in the field of healthcare in 2010 by earning a certificate in Plant-Based Nutrition through the T. Colin Campbell Foundation and eCornell University.

Dr. Rudolph has become an expert in nutrition and lifestyle medicine. He uses his expertise as an educator, speaker, and writer to help others learn how to prevent and reverse chronic disease by adopting a whole foods, plant-based lifestyle.

Notes

Introduction

1 IMS Institute for Healthcare Informatics. The Use of Medicines in the United States: Review of 2011. April 2012.

2 Centers for Disease Control. National Ambulatory Medical Care Survey: 2009 Summary Tables. Available at: http://www.cdc.gov/nchs/data/ahcd/namcs_summary/2009_namcs_web_tables.pdf. Accessed Feb 23, 2013.

3 Epstein AJ, et al. Coronary revascularization trends in the United States, 2001-2008. 2011 May 4;305(17):1769-1776.

4 Centers for Medicare and Medicaid Services, Office of the Actuary, National Health Statistics Group, National Health Expenditure Data. Available at: http://www.cms.gov/Research-Statistics-Data-and-Systems/Statistics-Trends-and-Reports/NationalHealthExpendData/NHE-Fact-Sheet.html. Accessed Feb 23, 2013.

Chapter 1 - Avoid the Pill Trap

1 IMS Institute for Healthcare Informatics. The Use of Medicines in the United States: Review of 2010. April 2011.

2 World Health Organization. World Health Statistics 2011. Available: http://www.who.int/whosis/whostat. Accessed July 5, 2011.

3 Centers for Disease Control and U.S. National Center for Health Statistics. Leading Causes of Death 1900-1998. Available: http://www.cdc.gov/nchs/data/statab/lead1900_98.pdf. Accessed July 5, 2011.

4 Centers for Disease Control and Prevention. National Diabetes Fact Sheet: national estimates and general information on diabetes and prediabetes in the United States, 2011. Atlanta, GA: U.S. Department of Health and Human Services, Centers for Disease Control and Prevention, 2011.

5 Boyle JP, Thompson TJ, Gregg EW, et al. Projection of the year 2050 burden of diabetes in the US adult population: dynamic modeling of incidence, mortality, and prediabetes prevalence. Popul Health Metr. 2010;8:29.

6   U.S. Cancer Statistics Working Group. United States Cancer Statistics: 1999–2007 Incidence and Mortality Web-based Report. Atlanta: U.S. Department of Health and Human Services, Centers for Disease Control and Prevention and National Cancer Institute; 2010.

Chapter 2 - Lose Weight, Gain Health, Eat as Much as You Want

1   Levi J, Segal L, St. Laurent R, Kohn D. F as in Fat: 2011 How Obesity Threatens America's Future. Trust For America's Health and The Robert Wood Johnson Foundation. July 2011.

2   Fuhrman J, Sarter B, Glaser D, et al. Changing perceptions of hunger on a high nutrient density diet. Nutr J. 2010 Nov 7;9:51.

3   NIH, NHLBI Obesity Education Initiative. Clinical Guidelines on the Identification, Evaluation, and Treatment of Overweight and Obesity in Adults. Available: http://www.nhlbi.nih.gov/guidelines/obesity/ob_gdlns.pdf.

4   National Institute of Diabetes and Digestive and Kidney Diseases (NIDDK). "Do You Know The Health Risks of Being Overweight?" U.S. Department of Health and Human Services. Available: http://win.niddk.nih.gov/publications/health_risks.htm. Accessed July 11, 2011.

5   Wang Y, Chen X, Song Y, et al. Association between obesity and kidney disease: A systematic review and meta-analysis. Kidney International. 2008 Jan 1;73:19-33.

6   Krauss RM, Winston M, Fletcher BJ, et al. Obesity Impact on Cardiovascular Disease. Circulation. 1998;98:1472-1476.

7   National Heart, Lung, and Blood Institute. "What Are the Health Risks of Overweight and Obesity?" Available: http://www.nhlbi.nih.gov/health/dci/Diseases/obe/obe_risks.html. Accessed July 11, 2011.

8   World Health Organization. Waist Circumference and Waist–Hip Ratio: Report of a WHO Expert Consultation. Publication Date - 2011. Geneva, 8-11 December 2008.

9   U.S. Department of Agriculture, Agricultural Research Service. 2012. Energy Intakes: Percentages of Energy from Protein, Carbohydrate, Fat, and Alcohol, by Gender and Age, *What We Eat in America*, NHANES 2009-2010. Available: www.ars.usda.gov/ba/bhnrc/fsrg. Accessed Feb 9, 2013.

10 Lobb A. Hepatoxicity associated with weight-loss supplements: A case for better post-marketing surveillance. World J Gastroenterol. 2009 April 14;15(14):1786–1787.

11 Wing RR, Phelan S. Long-term weight loss maintenance. American Journal of Clinical Nutrition. 2005 Jul;82(1):222S-225S.

12 Saris W. Very-Low-Calorie Diets and Sustained Weight Loss. Obesity Research. 2001;9:s295–s301.

13 Campbell TC, Campbell II TM. The China Study. Dallas, TX: Benbella Books, Inc. 2006.

14 Spencer EA, Appleby PN, et al. Diet and body mass index in 38000 EPIC-Oxford meat-eaters, fish-eaters, vegetarians and vegans. Int J Obes Relat Metab Disord. 2003 Jun;27(6):728-34.

15 Rosell M, Appleby P, et al. Weight gain over 5 years in 21,966 meat-eating, fish-eating, vegetarian, and vegan men and women in EPIC-Oxford. Int J Obes (Lond). 2006 Sep;30(9):1389-96.

16 Campbell TC, Chen J. Energy balance: interpretation of data from rural China. Toxicol Sci. 1999;52(1):87-94.

17 Wang S, Quan J, et al. Asian Americans and Obesity in California: A Protective Effect of Biculturalism. J Immigr Minor Health. 2011 April;13(2):276–283.

18 Goel MS, McCarthy EP, Phillips RS, Wee CC. Obesity among US immigrant subgroups by duration of residence. JAMA. 2004;292(23):2860.

19 Harris KA, Kris-Etherton PM. Effects of whole grains on coronary heart disease risk. Curr Atheroscler Rep. 2010 Nov;12(6):368-76.

20 Anderson JW, Baird P, et al. Health benefits of dietary fiber. Nutr Rev. 2009 Apr;67(4):188-205.

21 Papathanasopoulos A, Camilleri M. Dietary fiber supplements: effects in obesity and metabolic syndrome and relationship to gastrointestinal functions. Gastroenterology. 2010 Jan;138(1):65-72.e1-2. doi: 10.1053/j.gastro.2009.11.045. Epub 2009 Nov 18. Review.

22 Farmer B, Larson BT, et al. A vegetarian dietary pattern as a nutrient-dense approach to weight management: an analysis of the national health and nutrition examination survey 1999-2004. J Am Diet Assoc. 2011 Jun;111(6):819-27.

23 Mathers CD,Bernard C, Iburg KM, et al. Global Burden of Disease: data sources, methods and results. World Health Organization (WHO). 2004. Available: http://www.who.int/healthinfo/bod/en/index.html.

24 Sinatra ST, DeMarco J. Free radicals, oxidative stress, oxidized low density lipoprotein (LDL), and the heart: antioxidants and other strategies to limit cardiovascular damage. Conn Med. 1995 Oct;59(10):579-88.

25 Mathers CD,Bernard C, Iburg KM, et al. Global Burden of Disease: data sources, methods and results. World Health Organization (WHO). 2004. Available: http://www.who.int/healthinfo/bod/en/index.html.

26 Mathers CD,Bernard C, Iburg KM, et al. Global Burden of Disease: data sources, methods and results. World Health Organization (WHO). 2004. Available: http://www.who.int/healthinfo/bod/en/index.html.

27 Turner-McGrievy GM, Barnard ND, Scialli AR. A two-year randomized weight loss trial comparing a vegan diet to a more moderate low-fat diet. Obesity (Silver Spring). 2007 Sep;15(9):2276-81.

28 Farmer, Bonnie, "Comparison of nutrient intakes for vegetarians, non-vegetarians, and dieters : results from the National Health and Nutrition Examination Survey 1999-2004" (2009). Masters Theses and Doctoral Dissertations. Paper 150. Available: http://commons.emich.edu/theses/150.

29 Berkow S, Barnard N, Ferdowsian H. Vegetarian Diets and Weight Status. Nutr Rev. 2006 Apr;64(4):175-88.

Chapter 3 - Healthy Hearts

1 WHO. World health statistics 2009. Geneva: World Health Organization; 2009e.

2   Centers for Disease Control and Prevention. Compressed mortality file: underlying cause of death, 1979 to 2007. Atlanta, Ga: Centers for Disease Control and Prevention. Available: http://wonder.cdc.gov/mortSQl.html. Accessed Feb 12, 2012.

3   Roger VL, Go AS, Lloyd-Jones DM, et al. Heart Disease and Stroke Statistics—2012 Update: A Report From the American Heart Association. Circulation. 2012 Jan 3;125(1):e2-e220.

4   United States Department of Health and Human Services. The Greatest Pandemic: The United States in 1918-1919. Available: http://1918.pandemicflu.gov/the_pandemic. Accessed Feb 12 2012.

5   Texas Heart Institute. Heart anatomy. Available: http://www.texasheartinstitute.org/HIC/Anatomy/anatomy2.cfm. Accessed Feb 20, 2012.

6   Alberts B, Johnson A, Lewis J, et al. Molecular Biology of the Cell. 4th edition. New York: Garland Science; 2002.

7   Flam BR, Eichler DC, Solomonson LP. Endothelial nitric oxide production is tightly coupled to the citrulline-NO cycle. Nitric Oxide. 2007 Nov-Dec;17(3-4):115-21.

8   Förstermann U, Nakane M, Tracey WR, Pollock JS. Isoforms of nitric oxide synthase: functions in the cardiovascular system. Eur Heart J. 1993 Nov;14 Suppl I:10-5. Review.

9   Chockalingam A. World Hypertension Day and global awareness. Can J Cardiol. 2008 Jun;24(6):441-4. Review.

10 Egan BM, Zhao Y, Axon RN. US Trends in Prevalence, Awareness, Treatment, and Control of Hypertension, 1988-2008. JAMA. 2010;303(20):2043-2050.

11 Zalewski A, Shi Y, Johnson AG. Diverse origin of intimal cells: smooth muscle cells, myofibroblasts, fibroblasts, and beyond? Circ Res. 2002;91:652-5.

12 Wolf C, Cai WJ, Vosschulte R, Kolati S, et al. Vascular remodeling and altered protein expression during growth of coronary collateral arteries. J Mol Cell Cardiol. 1998;30:2291-305.

13 Astrup A, Dyerberg J, Elwood P, et al. The role of reducing intakes of saturated fat in the prevention of cardiovascular disease: where does the evidence stand in 2010? Am J Clin Nutr. 2011 Apr;93(4):684-688.

14 Frink RJ. Inflammatory Atherosclerosis: Characteristics of the Injurious Agent. Sacramento (CA): Heart Research Foundation; 2002.

15 Slevin M, Krupinski J, Badimon L. Controlling the angiogenic switch in developing atherosclerotic plaques: possible targets for therapeutic intervention. J Angiogenes Res. 2009 Sep 21;1:4.

16 Rudijanto A. The role of vascular smooth muscle cells on the pathogenesis of atherosclerosis. Acta Med Ind-Ind J Int Med. 2007 Apr-Jun;39(2):86-93.

17 Hirst DG, Robson T. Nitric Oxide Physiology and Pathology. Methods Mol Biol. 2011;704:1-13. Review.

18 Badimon L, Storey RF, Vilahur G. Update on lipids, inflammation and atherothrombosis. Thromb Haemost. 2011 May;105 Suppl 1:S34-42.

19 McGill, Jr. HC, McMahan CA, Herderick EE, et al. Origin of atherosclerosis in childhood and adolescence. Am J Clin Nutr. 2000 Nov;72(5):1307S-1315s.

20 Chandrasekaran B, Kurbaan AS. Myocardial infarction with angiographically normal coronary arteries. J R Soc Med. 2002 August;95(8):398–400.

21 Macrez R, Ali C, Toutirais O, et al. Stroke and the immune system: from pathophysiology to new therapeutic strategies. Lancet Neurol. 2011 May;10(5):471-480. Review.

22 Falk E. Pathogenesis of Atherosclerosis. J Am Coll Cardiol, 2006;47:7-12.

23 Boden WE, O'Rourke RA, Teo KK, et al. Optimal medical therapy with or without PCI for stable coronary disease. N Engl J Med. 2007 Apr 12;356(15): 1503-16.

24 Peduzzi P, Kamina A, Detre K. Twenty-two-year follow-up in the VA Cooperative Study of Coronary Artery Bypass Surgery for Stable Angina. Am J Cardiol. 1998 Jun 15;81(12):1393-9.

25 Reichenberg A, Dahlman KL, Mosovich S, Silverstein JH. Neuropsychiatric consequences of coronary artery bypass grafting and noncardiovascular surgery. Dialogues Clin Neurosci. 2007;9(1):85-91. Review.

26 Esselstyn, Jr. CB. Prevent and Reverse Heart Disease. New York, NY: Penguin Group (USA) Inc. 2007.

27 Roberts WC. Twenty questions on atherosclerosis. Proc (Bayl Univ Med Cent). 2000 April;13(2):139-143.

28 Esselstyn CB Jr. Updating a 12-year experience with arrest and reversal therapy for coronary heart disease (an overdue requiem for palliative cardiology). Am J Cardiol. 1999 Aug 1;84(3):339-41,A8.

29 Vrecer M, Turk S, Drinovec J, Mrhar A. Use of statins in primary and secondary prevention of coronary heart disease and ischemic stroke. Meta-analysis of randomized trials. Int J Clin Pharmacol Ther. 2003 Dec;41(12):567-77.

30 Newman, D. Statin drugs given for 5 years for heart disease prevention (without known heart disease). theNNT. 2013 Nov 2. Available: http://www.thennt.com/nnt/statins-for-heart-disease-prevention-without-prior-heart-disease/. Accessed Nov 24, 2013.

31 Newman, D. Statins given for 5 years for heart disease prevention (with known heart disease). theNNT. 2013 Nov 2. Available: http://www.thennt.com/nnt/statins-for-heart-disease-prevention-with-known-heart-disease/. Accessed Nov 24, 2013.

32 S. Sultan and N. Hynes, "The Ugly Side of Statins. Systemic Appraisal of the Contemporary Un-Known Unknowns," Open Journal of Endocrine and Metabolic Diseases, Vol. 3 No. 3, 2013, pp. 179-185. doi: 10.4236/ojemd.2013.33025.

33 Rennison JH, Van Wagoner DR. Impact of Dietary Fatty Acids on Cardiac Arrhythmogenesis. Circulation: Arrhythmia and Electrophysiology. 2009;2:460-469.

34 Heeringa J, van der Kuip DA, Hofman A, et al. Subclinical atherosclerosis and risk of atrial fibrillation: The Rotterdam Study. Arch Intern Med. 2007 Feb 26;167(4):382-7.

35 Djoussé L, Rautaharju PM, Hopkins PN, et al. Dietary linolenic acid and adjusted QT and JT intervals in the National Heart, Lung, and Blood Institute Family Heart study. J Am Coll Cardiol. 2005 May 17;45(10):1716-22.

36 Burdge GC, Finnegan YE, Minihane AM, et al. Effect of altered dietary n-3 fatty acid intake upon plasma lipid fatty acid composition, conversion of [13C]alpha-linolenic acid to longer-chain fatty acids and partitioning towards beta-oxidation in older men. Br J Nutr. 2003 Aug;90(2):311-21.

37 Virtanen JK, Laukkanen JA, Mursu J, et al. Serum Long-Chain n-3 Poly-unsaturated Fatty Acids, Mercury, and Risk of Sudden Cardiac Death in Men: A Prospective Population-Based Study. PLoS One. 2012;7(7):e41046. Epub 2012 Jul 16.

38 Albert CM, Oh K, Whang W, et al. Dietary α-Linolenic Acid Intake and Risk of Sudden Cardiac Death and Coronary Heart Disease Circulation. 2005;112:3232-3238.

39 Tapiero H, Mathé G, Couvreur P, Tew KD. I. Arginine. Biomed Pharmacother. 2002 Nov;56(9):439-45. Review.

40 Visek WJ. Arginine needs, physiological states and usual diets: A reevaluation. J. Nutr. 1986 Jan 1;116(1):36-46.

Chapter 4 - Winning the Battle Against Type 2 Diabetes

1 Centers for Disease Control and Prevention. National diabetes fact sheet: national estimates and general information on diabetes and prediabetes in the United States, 2011. Atlanta, GA: U.S. Department of Health and Human Services, Centers for Disease Control and Prevention, 2011.

2 Kolditz CI, Langin D. Adipose tissue lipolysis. Current Opinion in Clin Nutr & Metabolic Care. 2010 Jul;13(4):377-381.

3 Lelliott C, Vidal-Puig AJ. Lipotoxicity, an imbalance between lipogenesis de novo and fatty acid oxidation. Int J Obes Relat Metab Disord. 2004 Dec;28 Suppl 4:S22-8.

4 Unger RH, Orci L. Lipotoxic diseases of nonadipose tissues in obesity. Int J Obes Relat Metab Disord. 2000 Nov;24(4):S28-S32.

5 Eckardt K, Taube A, Eckel J. Obesity-associated insulin resistance in skeletal muscle: role of lipid accumulation and physical inactivity. Rev Endocr Metab Disord. 2011 Sep;12(3):163-72.

6 Ezaki O. Regulatory Elements in the Insulin-Responsive Glucose Transporter (GLUT4) Gene. Biochem and Biophys Res Comm. 1997 Dec;241(1):1-6.

7 Foufelle F, Ferré P. New perspectives in the regulation of hepatic glycolytic and lipogenic genes by insulin and glucose: a role for the transcription factor sterol regulatory element binding protein-1c. Biochem J. 2002 September 1;366 (Pt 2):377–391.

8 Aguer C, Mercier J, et al. Intramyocellular lipid accumulation is associated with permanent relocation ex vivo and in vitro of fatty acid translocase (FAT)/CD36 in obese patients. Diabetologia. 2010;53:1151-1163.

9 Moro C, Galgani JE, Luu L, et al. Influence of gender, obesity, and muscle lipase activity on intramyocellular lipids in sedentary individuals. J Clin Endocrinol Metab. 2009;94:3440-3447.

10 Adams JM, Pratipanawatr T, Berria R. et al. Ceramide content is increased in skeletal muscle from obese insulin-resistant humans. Diabetes. 2004;53:25-31.

11 Alkhateeb H, Chabowski A, Glatz JF, et al. Restoring AS160 phosphorylation rescues skeletal muscle insulin resistance and fatty acid oxidation while not reducing intramuscular lipids. Am J Physiol Endocrinol Metab. 2009 Nov;297(5):E1056-66.

12 Shoelson SE, Lee J, Yaun M. Inflammation and the IKK beta/I kappa B/NF-kappa B axis in obesity- and diet-induced insulin resistance. Int J Obes Relat Metab Disord. 2003 Dec;27 Suppl 3:S49-52.

13 Puigserver P, Wu Z, Park CW, et al. A cold-inducible coactivator of nuclear receptors linked to adaptive thermogenesis. Cell. 1998 Mar 20;92(6):829-39.

14 Voet, D, Voet JG, Pratt CW. Fundamentals of Biochemistry, 2nd Edition. 2006. John Wiley and Sons, Inc.. pp. 547.

15 Patti MF, Butte AJ, Crunkhorn S, et al. Coordinated reduction of genes of oxidative metabolism in humans with insulin resistance and diabetes: Potential role of PGC-1 and NRF1. Proc Natl Acad Sci USA. 2003;100:8466-8471.

16 Mootha VK, Lindgren CM, Eriksson KF, et al. PGC-1 alpha-responsive genes involved in oxidative phosphorylation are coordinately down regulated in human diabetes. Nat Genet. 2003;34:267-273.

17 Hemmingsen B, Lund SS, et al. Targeting intensive glycaemic control versus targeting conventional glycaemic control for type 2 diabetes mellitus. Cochrane Database of Systematic Reviews 2013, Issue 11. Art. No.: CD008143. DOI: 10.1002/14651858.CD008143.pub3.

18 Mazzola N. Review of current and emerging therapies in type 2 diabetes mellitus. Am J Manag Care. 2012 Jan;18(1 Suppl):S17-26. Review.

19 Currie CJ, Poole CD, Evans M, et al. Mortality and other important diabetes-related outcomes with insulin vs other antihyperglycemic therapies in type 2 diabetes. J Clin Endocrinol Metab. 2013 Feb;98(2):668-77. doi: 10.1210/jc.2012-3042.

20 Quianzon CC, Cheikh IE. History of current non-insulin medications for diabetes mellitus. J Community Hosp Intern Med Perspect. 2012 Oct 15;2(3). doi: 10.3402/jchimp.v2i3.19081. Print 2012.

21 Djoussé L, Gaziano JM, Buring JE, Lee IM. Dietary omega-3 fatty acids and fish consumption and risk of type 2 diabetes. Am J Clin Nutr. 2011 Jan; 93(1):143-50.

22 Eilat-Adar S, Xu J, et al. Adherence to Dietary Recommendations for Saturated Fat, Fiber, and Sodium Is Low in American Indians and Other U.S. Adults with Diabetes. J. Nutr. 2008 Sept 1;138(9):1699-1704.

23 Morgan NG. Fatty acids and [beta]-cell toxicity. Curr Opin Clin Nut Met Care. 2009 Mar;12(2):117-122.

24 Wolfram T, Ismail-Beigi F. Efficacy of high-fiber diets in the management of type 2 diabetes mellitus. Endocr Pract. 2011 Jan-Feb;17(1):132-42.

25 Physicians Committee For Responsible Medicine. NutritionMD recipes. Available: http://www.nutritionmd.org/. Accessed Mar 20, 2012.

26 American Diabetes Association. Food & Fitness recipes. Available: http://www.diabetes.org/. Accessed Mar 20, 2012.

27 Jing HE, Goodpaster BH, Kelley DE. Effects of Weight Loss and Physical Activity on Muscle Lipid Content and Droplet Size. Obesity Research. 2004;12:761-769.

28 Toledo FG, Menshikova EV, Ritov VB, et al. Effects of Physical Activity and Weight Loss on Skeletal Muscle Mitochondria and Relationship With Glucose Control in Type 2 Diabetes. Diabetes. 2007 Aug;56(8):2142-2147.

29 Eckardt K, Taube A, Eckel J. Obesity-associated insulin resistance in skeletal muscle: Role of lipid accumulation and physical inactivity. Rev Endocr Metab Disord. 2011 Feb;published online ahead of print. DOI:10.1007/s11154-011-9168-2.

30 Lin J, Wu H, Tarr PT, et al. Transcriptional co-activator PGC-1 alpha drives the formation of slow-twitch muscle fibres. Nature. 2002 Aug;418:797-801.

Chapter 5 - A Cancer-Free Life—Is It Possible?

1 Blendon RJ, Benson JM, Weldon KJ. Five-Country Alzheimer's Disease Survey. Harvard School of Public Health and Alzheimer Europe. 2011 Feb.

2 Mathers CD, Boerma T, Ma Fat D. Global and regional causes of death. Br Med Bull. 2009;92:7-32. Epub. Review.

3 Beaglehole R, Bonita R, Magnusson R. Global cancer prevention: an important pathway to global health and development. Public Health. 2011 Dec; 125(12):821-31. Review.

4 Sindayikengera S, Wen-shui X. Nutritional evaluation of caseins and whey proteins and their hydrolysates from Protamex J Zhejiang Univ Sci B. 2006 February;7(2):90–98.

5 Madhavan TV, Gopalan C. The effect of dietary protein on carcinogenesis of aflatoxin. Arch Pathol. 1968 Feb;85(2):133-7.

6 Appleton BS, Campbell TC. Inhibition of aflatoxin-initiated preneoplastic liver lesions by low dietary protein. Nutr Cancer. 1982;3(4):200-6.

7 Dunaif GE, Campbell TC. Dietary protein level and aflatoxin B1-induced preneoplastic hepatic lesions in the rat. J Nutr. 1987 Jul;117(7):1298-302.

8 Schulsinger DA, Root MM, Campbell TC. Effect of Dietary Protein Quality on Development of Aflatoxin B1-Induced Hepatic Preneoplastic Lesions. J Natl Cancer Inst. 1989;81(16):1241-1245.

9 Campbell TC, Campbell II TM. The China Study. Dallas, TX: Benbella Books, Inc. 2006.

10 van der Pols JC, Bain C, Gunnell D, et al. Childhood dairy intake and adult cancer risk: 65-y follow-up of the Boyd Orr cohort. Am J Clin Nutr. 2007 Dec;86(6):1722-1729.

11 Chan JM, Giovannucci E, Andersson SO, et al. Dairy products, calcium, phosphorous, vitamin D, and risk of prostate cancer (Sweden) Cancer Causes Control. 1998 Dec;9(6):559-66.

12 American Cancer Society: Estimated Number of New Cancer Cases and Deaths by Sex, US, 2013. Available: http://www.cancer.org/acs/groups/content/@epidemiologysurveilance/documents/document/acspc-037124.pdf. Accessed Dec 12, 2013.

13 Key TJ, Appleby PN, Spencer EA, et al. Cancer incidence in vegetarians: results from the European Prospective Investigation into Cancer and Nutrition (EPIC-Oxford). Am J Clin Nutr. 2009 May;89(5):1620S-1626S.

14 Tonstad S, Butler T, Yan R, Fraser GE. Type of vegetarian diet, body weight, and prevalence of type 2 diabetes. Diabetes Care. 2009 May;32(5):791-6.

15 Khandekar MJ, Cohen P, Spiegelman BM. Molecular mechanisms of cancer development in obesity. Nat Rev Cancer. 2011 Nov 24;11(12):886-95.

16 World Cancer Research Fund/American Institute for Cancer Research. Food, nutrition, physical activity, and the prevention of cancer: a global perspective. Washington DC: AICR; 2007. pp. 22–25.

17 Lanou AJ, Svenson B. Reduced cancer risk in vegetarians: an analysis of recent reports. Cancer Manag Res. 2011;3:1–8.

18 Turesky RJ. Formation and biochemistry of carcinogenic heterocyclic aromatic amines in cooked meats. Toxicol Lett. 2007 Feb 5;168(3):219-27.

19 Richman EL, Stampfer MJ, Paciorek A, et al. Intakes of meat, fish, poultry, and eggs and risk of prostate cancer progression. Am J Clin Nutr. 2010 Mar;91(3):712-21.

20 Hanahan D, Folkman J. Patterns and emerging mechanisms of the angiogenic switch during tumorigenesis. Cell. 1996 Aug 9;86(3):353-64. Review.

21 Rak J, Mitsuhashi Y, Bayko L, et al. Mutant ras Oncogenes Upregulate VEGF/VPF Expression: Implications for Induction and Inhibition of Tumor Angiogenesis Cancer Res. 15 Oct 1995;55:4575.

22 Li WW. "Can we eat to starve cancer?" TED2010. Feb 2010. Available: http://www.ted.com/talks/william_li.html. Accessed Apr 15, 2012.

23 Li WW, Li VW, Hutnik M, et al. Tumor Angiogenesis as a Target for Dietary Cancer Prevention. J Oncology. Volume 2012 (2012), Article ID 879623, 23 pages, doi:10.1155/2012/879623.

24 Bertram JS. The molecular biology of cancer. Mol Aspects Med. 2000 Dec;21(6):167-223. Review.

25 Calvo MB, Figueroa A, Pulido EG, et al. Potential role of sugar transporters in cancer and their relationship with anticancer therapy. Int J Endocrinol. 2010;2010. pii: 205357.

26 Lopez-Rios F, Sanchez-Arago M, Garcia-Garcia E, et al. Loss of the mitochondrial bioenergetics capacity underlies the glucose avidity of carcinomas. Cancer Res. 2007;67:9013–9017. doi:10.1158/0008-5472.CAN-07-1678.

27 Young CD, Anderson SM. Sugar and fat - that's where it's at: metabolic changes in tumors. Breast Cancer Res. 2008;10(1):202. Review.

28 Jaye A, Merzer G. Unprocessed. Hail to the Kale Publishing. 2011.

29 Neklason DW, Thorpe BL, Ferrandez A, et al. Colonic adenoma risk in familial colorectal cancer—a study of six extended kindreds. Am J Gastroenterol. 2008 Oct;103(10):2577-84.

Chapter 6 - Autoimmune Diseases

1 Karopka T, Fluck J, Mevissen HT, et al. The Autoimmune Disease Database: a dynamically compiled literature-derived database. BMC Bioinformatics. 2006 Jun 27;7:325.

2 Pugliatti M, Sotgiu S, Rosati G. The worldwide prevalence of multiple sclerosis. Clin Neurol Neurosurg. 2002;104:182–91.

3 Sicotte NL. Neuroimaging in multiple sclerosis: neurotherapeutic implications. Neurotherapeutics. 2011 Jan;8(1):54-62. Review.

4 Korn T. Pathophysiology of multiple sclerosis. J Neurol. 2008 Dec;255 Suppl 6:2-6. Review.

5 Scalfari A, Neuhaus A, Degenhardt A, et al. The natural history of multiple sclerosis: a geographically based study 10: relapses and long-term disability. Brain. 2010 Jul;133(Pt 7):1914-29.

6 Goldberg LD, Edwards NC, Fincher C, et al. Comparing the cost-effectiveness of disease-modifying drugs for the first-line treatment of relapsing-remitting multiple sclerosis. J Manag Care Pharm. 2009 Sep;15(7):543-55.

7 Kappos L, Freedman MS, Polman CH, et al. Long-term effect of early treatment with interferon beta-1b after a first clinical event suggestive of multiple sclerosis: 5-year active treatment extension of the phase 3 BENEFIT trial. Lanc Neuro. 2009 Nov;8(11):987-997.

8 Pizza Hut. Nutritional information: pizza. Available: www.pizzahut.com/nutritionpizza.html. Accessed: May 14, 2012.

9 Swank RL, Dugan BB. Effect of low saturated fat diet in early and late cases of multiple sclerosis. Lancet. 1990 Jul 7;336(8706):37-9.

10 Goodin DS, Reder AT, Ebers GC, et al. Survival in MS: A randomized cohort study 21 years after the start of the pivotal IFNß-1b trial. Neurology. 2012 Apr 24;78(17):1315-22.

11 Munger KL, Chitnis T, Frazier AL, et al. Dietary intake of vitamin D during adolescence and risk of multiple sclerosis. J Neurol. 2011 Mar; 258(3):479-85.

12 Michaud K, Wolfe F. Comorbidities in rheumatoid arthritis. Best Pract Res Clin Rheumatol. 2007 Oct;21(5):885-906. Review.

13 van der Kooij SM, de Vries-Bouwstra JK, Goekoop-Ruiterman YP, et al. Limited efficacy of conventional DMARDs after initial methotrexate failure in patients with recent onset rheumatoid arthritis treated according to the disease activity score. Ann Rheum Dis. 2007 Oct;66(10):1356-62.

14 Galindo-Rodriguez G, Aviña-Zubieta JA, Russell AS, Suarez-Almazor ME. Disappointing long-term results with disease modifying antirheumatic drugs. A practice based study. J Rheumatol. 1999 Nov;26(11):2337-43.

15 Attar SM. Adverse effects of low dose methotrexate in rheumatoid arthritis patients. A hospital-based study. Saudi Med J. 2010 Aug;31(8):909-15.

16 AHFS Consumer Medication Information. Methotrexate. U.S. National Library of Medicine. Available: http://www.ncbi.nlm.nih.gov/pubmedhealth/ PMH0000547/. Accessed: May 15, 2012.

17 Da Silva JA, Jacobs JW, Kirwan JR, et al. Safety of low dose glucocorticoid treatment in rheumatoid arthritis: published evidence and prospective trial data. Ann Rheum Dis. 2006 Mar;65(3):285-93.

18 Doan QV, Chiou CF, Dubois RW. Review of eight pharmacoeconomic studies of the value of biologic DMARDs (adalimumab, etanercept, and infiximab) in the management of rheumatoid arthritis. J Manag Care Pharm. 2006;12(7):555-69.

19 Leombruno JP, Einarson TR, Keystone EC. The safety of anti-tumour necrosis factor treatments in rheumatoid arthritis: meta and exposure-adjusted pooled analyses of serious adverse events. Ann Rheum Dis. 2009 Jul;68(7):1136-45.

20 Curtis JR, Xie F, Chen L, et al. The comparative risk of serious infections among rheumatoid arthritis patients starting or switching biological agents. Ann Rheum Dis. 2011 Aug;70(8):1401-6.

21 Fuhrman J, Sarter B, Calabro DJ. Brief case reports of medically supervised, water-only fasting associated with remission of autoimmune disease. Alt Ther. 2002 Jul/Aug;8(4):112,110-1.

22 Müller H, de Toledo FW, Resch KL. Fasting followed by vegetarian diet in patients with rheumatoid arthritis: a systematic review. Scand J Rheumatol. 2001;30(1):1-10. Review.

23 Haugen M, Fraser D, et al. Diet therapy for the patient with rheumatoid arthritis? Rheumatology. 1999;38(11):1039-1044.

24 D'Cruz DP. Systemic lupus erythematosus. BMJ. 2006 April 15;332(7546): 890–894.

25 Roman MJ, Shanker BA, Davis A, et al. Prevalence and correlates of accelerated atherosclerosis in systemic lupus erythematosus. N Engl J Med. 2003 Dec 18;349(25):2399-406. Erratum in: N Engl J Med. 2006 Oct 19;355(16):1746.

26 Molokhia M, McKeigue P. Systemic lupus erythematosus: genes versus environment in high risk populations. Lupus. 2006;15(11):827-32. Review.

27 Arbuckle MR, McClain MT, Rubertone MV, et al. Development of autoantibodies before the clinical onset of systemic lupus erythematosus. N Engl J Med. 2003 Oct 16;349(16):1526-33.

28 Yildirim-Toruner C, Diamond B. Current and novel therapeutics in the treatment of systemic lupus erythematosus. J Allergy Clin Immunol. 2011 Feb;127(2): 303-12; quiz 313-4. Review.

29 Morand EF, McCloud PI, Littlejohn GO. Continuation of long term treatment with hydroxychloroquine in systemic lupus erythematosus and rheumatoid arthritis. Ann Rheum Dis. 1992 Dec;51(12):1318–1321.

30 Postal M, Costallat L, Appenzeller S. Biological Therapy in Systemic Lupus Erythematosus. Int J Rheum. 2012;2012:578641.

31 Trager J, Ward MM. Mortality and causes of death in systemic lupus erythematosus. Curr Opi Rheum. 2001 Sept;13(5):345-351.

32 Fuhrman J, Sarter B, Calabro DJ. Brief case reports of medically supervised, water-only fasting associated with remission of autoimmune disease. Alt Ther. 2002 Jul/Aug;8(4):112,110-1.

33 Brown AC. Lupus erythematosus and nutrition: a review of the literature. J Ren Nutr. 2000 Oct;10(4):170-83. Review.

34 Hancock L, Windsor AC, Mortensen NJ. Inflammatory bowel disease: the view of the surgeon. Colorectal Dis. 2006 May;8 Suppl 1:10-4. Review.

35 Tamboli CP, Neut C, Desreumaux P, Colombel JF. Dysbiosis in inflammatory bowel disease. Gut. 2004;53:1–4.

36 Chiba M, Toru A, Hidehiko T, et al. Lifestyle-related disease in Crohn's disease: Relapse prevention by a semi-vegetarian diet. World J Gastroenterol. 2010 May 28;16(20):2484–2495.

37 Pardasani AG, Feldman SR, Clark AR. Treatment of Psoriasis: An Algorithm-Based Approach for Primary Care Physicians. Am Fam Physician. 2000 Feb 1;61(3):725-733.

38 Gelfand JM, Gladman DD, Mease PJ, et al. Epidemiology of psoriatic arthritis in the population of the United States. J Am Acad Dermatol. 2005 Oct;53(4):573.

39 Lebwohl M, Ting PT, Koo JY. Psoriasis treatment: traditional therapy. Ann Rheum Dis. 2005 Mar;64 Suppl 2:ii83-6. Review.

40 Heller MM, Lee ES, Koo JY. Stress as an influencing factor in psoriasis. Skin Therapy Lett. 2011 May;16(5):1-4.

41 Wolters M. Diet and psoriasis: experimental data and clinical evidence. Br J Dermatol. 2005 Oct;153(4):706-14. Review.

Chapter 7 - The Rest of the Story: Healthy Skin, Eyes, Kidneys, and Brain

1 Kanitakis J. Anatomy, histology and immunohistochemistry of normal human skin. Eur J Dermatol. 2002 Jul-Aug;12(4):390-9; quiz 400-1. Review.

2 Lee SH, Jeong SK, Ahn SK. An update of the defensive barrier function of skin. Yonsei Med J. 2006 Jun 30;47(3):293-306. Review.

3 Marks JG, Miller J. Lookingbill and Marks' Principles of Dermatology (4th ed.). 2006. Elsevier. pp. 1-9.

4 Morita A. Tobacco smoke causes premature skin aging. J Dermatol Sci. 2007 Dec;48(3):169-75.

5 Sanders CS, Chang H, Salzmann S, et al. Photoaging is associated with protein oxidation in human skin in vivo. J Invest Dermatol. 2002 Apr;118(4):618-25.

6 Nagata C, Nakamura K, Wada K, et al. Association of dietary fat, vegetables and antioxidant micronutrients with skin ageing in Japanese women. Br J Nutr. 2010 May;103(10):1493-8.

7 Bae JY, Lim SS, Kim SJ, et al. Bog blueberry anthocyanins alleviate photoaging in ultraviolet-B irradiation-induced human dermal fibroblasts. Mol Nutr Food Res. 2009 Jun;53(6):726-38.

8 Aslam MN, Lansky EP, Varani J. Pomegranate as a cosmeceutical source: pomegranate fractions promote proliferation and procollagen synthesis and inhibit matrix metalloproteinase-1 production in human skin cells. J Ethnopharmacol. 2006 Feb 20;103(3):311-8.

9 Byfield SD, Chen D, Yim YM, et al. Age distribution of patients with advanced non-melanoma skin cancer in the United States. Arch Dermatol Res. 2013; 305: 845–850.

10 Howlader N, Noone AM, Krapcho M, et al. SEER Cancer Statistics Review, 1975-2009 (Vintage 2009 Populations), National Cancer Institute. Bethesda, MD, http://seer.cancer.gov/csr/1975_2009_pops09/, based on November 2011 SEER data submission, posted to the SEER web site, 2012.

11 Shapira N. Nutritional approach to sun protection: a suggested complement to external strategies. Nutr Rev. 2010 Feb;68(2):75-86.

12 Sies H, Stahl W. Nutritional protection against skin damage from sunlight. Annu Rev Nutr. 2004;24:173-200.

13 Ibiebele TI, van der Pols JC, Hughes MC, et al. Dietary pattern in association with squamous cell carcinoma of the skin: a prospective study. Am J Clin Nutr. 2007 May;85(5):1401-8.

14 Samarasinghe V, Madan V. Nonmelanoma Skin Cancer. J Cutan Aesthet Surg. 2012 Jan-Mar;5(1):3–10.

15 Love WE, Bernhard JD, Bordeaux JS. Topical imiquimod or fluorouracil therapy for basal and squamous cell carcinoma: a systematic review. Arch Dermatol. 2009 Dec;145(12):1431-8. Review.

16 Appleby PN, Allen NE, Key TJ. Diet, vegetarianism, and cataract risk. Am J Clin Nutr. 2011 May;93(5):1128-35.

17 Appleby PN, Allen NE, Key TJ. Diet, vegetarianism, and cataract risk. Am J Clin Nutr. 2011 May;93(5):1128-35.

18 Everitt AV, Hilmer SN, Brand-Miller JC, et al. Dietary approaches that delay age-related diseases. Clin Interv Aging. 2006;1(1):11-31. Review.

19 Mares JA, Voland RP, Sondel SA, et al. Healthy lifestyles related to subsequent prevalence of age-related macular degeneration. Arch Ophthalmol. 2011 Apr;129(4):470-80.

20 Rabin RC. The reward for donating a kidney: No insurance. The New York Times. 11 Jun 2012.

21 Laliberté F, Bookhart BK, Vekeman F, et al. Direct all-cause health care costs associated with chronic kidney disease in patients with diabetes and hypertension: a managed care perspective. J Manag Care Pharm. 2009 May;15 (4):312-22.

22 Zhang QL, Rothenbacher D. Prevalence of chronic kidney disease in population-based studies: systematic review. BMC Public Health. 2008 Apr 11;8:117. Review.

23 Fulgoni VL 3rd. Current protein intake in America: analysis of the National Health and Nutrition Examination Survey, 2003-2004. Am J Clin Nutr. 2008 May;87(5):1554S-1557S.

24 Brenner BM, Meyer TW, Hostetter TH. Dietary protein intake and the progressive nature of kidney disease: the role of hemodynamically mediated glomerular injury in the pathogenesis of progressive glomerular sclerosis in aging, renal ablation, and intrinsic renal disease. N Engl J Med. 1982 Sep 9; 307(11):652-9. Review.

25 Lindeman RD. Changes in renal function with aging. Implications for treatment. Drugs Aging. 1992 Sep-Oct;2(5):423-31. Review.

26 Bernstein AM, Treyzon L, Li Z. Are high-protein, vegetable-based diets safe for kidney function? A review of the literature. J Am Diet Assoc. 2007 Apr;107(4):644-50. Review.

27 Barsotti G, Morelli E, Cupisti A, et al. A special, supplemented 'vegan' diet for nephrotic patients. Am J Nephrol. 1991;11(5):380-5.

28 Finkielstein VA, Goldfarb DS. Strategies for preventing calcium oxalate stones. CMAJ. 2006 May 9;174(10):1407-9.

29 Taylor EN, Fung TT, Curhan GC. DASH-style diet associates with reduced risk for kidney stones. J Am Soc Nephrol. 2009 Oct;20(10):2253-9.

30 Hoyert DL, Xu JQ. Deaths: Preliminary data for 2011. National vital statistics reports; vol 61 no 6. Hyattsville, MD: National Center for Health Statistics. 2012.

31 Xie J, Brayne C, Matthews FE, et al. Survival times in people with dementia: analysis from population based cohort study with 14 year follow-up. BMJ. 2008 Feb 2;336(7638):258-62.

32 Atri A. Effective pharmacological management of Alzheimer's disease. Am J Manag Care. 2011 Nov;17 Suppl 13:S346-55. Review.
33 Casey DA, Antimisiaris D, O'Brien J. Drugs for Alzheimer's disease: are they effective? P T. 2010 Apr;35(4):208-11.
34 Morris MC, Evans DA, Tangney CC, et al. Dietary copper and high saturated and trans fat intakes associated with cognitive decline. Arch Neurol. 2006 Aug;63(8):1085-8.
35 Kivipelto M, Helkala EL, Laakso MP, et al. Apolipoprotein E epsilon4 allele, elevated midlife total cholesterol level, and high midlife systolic blood pressure are independent risk factors for late-life Alzheimer disease. Ann Intern Med. 2002 Aug 6;137(3):149-55.
36 Notkola IL, Sulkava R, Pekkanen J, et al. Serum total cholesterol, apolipoprotein E epsilon 4 allele, and Alzheimer's disease. Neuroepidemiology. 1998;17(1):14-20.
37 Serrano-Pozo A, Frosch MP, Masliah E, Hyman BT. Neuropathological alterations in Alzheimer disease. Cold Spring Harb Perspect Biol. Sep 2011;3(9):a006189.
38 Koudinov AR, Koudinova NV. Brain cholesterol pathology is the cause of Alzheimer's disease. Clin Med Health Res. 2001:clinmed/2001100005.
39 Hughes TF, Andel R, Small BJ, et al. Midlife fruit and vegetable consumption and risk of dementia in later life in Swedish twins. Am J Geriatr Psychiatry. 2010 May;18(5):413-20.
40 Pasinetti GM, Wang J, Porter S, Ho L. Caloric intake, dietary lifestyles, macronutrient composition, and Alzheimer's disease dementia. Int J Alzheimers Dis. 2011;2011:806293.
41 Robson LG, Dyall S, Sidloff D, Michael-Titus AT. Omega-3 polyunsaturated fatty acids increase the neurite outgrowth of rat sensory neurones throughout development and in aged animals. Neurobiol Aging. 2010 Apr;31(4):678-87.
42 Lim GP, Calon F, Morihara T, et al. A diet enriched with the omega-3 fatty acid docosahexaenoic acid reduces amyloid burden in an aged Alzheimer mouse model. J Neurosci. 2005 Mar 23;25(12):3032-40.

Chapter 8 - A Look Behind the Scenes of Medicine, Food, and Politics

1 Noakes TD, Borresen J, Hew-Butler T, et al. Semmelweis and the aetiology of puerperal sepsis 160 years on: an historical review. Epidemiol Infect. 2008 Jan;136(1):1-9.
2 Ahmed N. 23 years of the discovery of Helicobacter pylori: Is the debate over? Ann Clin Microbiol Antimicrob. 2005;4:17.
3 Marshall B, Adams PC. Helicobacter pylori: A Nobel pursuit? Can J Gastroenterol. 2008 November;22(11):895–896.
4 Abbott, A. Medical Nobel awarded for ulcers: Discoverers of Helicobacter pylori earn medicine's highest honour. Nature. 3 Oct 2005. Available: http://www.nature.com/news/2005/051003/full/news051003-2.html. Accessed Dec 9, 2011.
5 Committee on Nutrition in Medical Education, Food and Nutrition Board, Council on Life Sciences, National Research Council. Nutrition Education in US Medical Schools. Washington, DC: National Academy Press; 1985.

6   Adams KM, Kohlmeier M, Zeisel SH. Nutrition education in U.S. medical schools: latest update of a national survey. Acad Med. 2010 Sep;85(9): 1537-42.

7   Frantz DJ, Munroe C, McClave SA, et al. Current perception of nutrition education in U.S. medical schools. Curr Gastroenterol Rep. 2011 Aug; 13(4):376-9. Review.

8   Lazarus K. Nutrition practices of family physicians after education by a physician nutrition specialist. Am J Clin Nutr. 1997 Jun;65(6 Suppl): 2007S-2009S.

9   Greger M. Nutrition education mandate introduced for doctors. 11 Nov 2011. Available: http://nutritionfacts.org/videos/nutrition-education-mandate-introduced-for-doctors/. Accessed Dec 10, 2011.

10 Greger M. Medical Associations oppose bill to mandate nutritional education. 14 Nov 2011. Available: http://nutritionfacts.org/videos/medical-associations-oppose-bill-to-mandate-nutrition-training/. Accessed Dec 10, 2011.

11 SB 380 Senate Bill (2011). Available: http://www.leginfo.ca.gov/pub/11-12/bill/sen/sb_0351-0400/sb_380_bill_20110906_chaptered.pdf. Accessed Dec 10, 2011.

12 Nguyen D, Ornstein C, Weber T. Dollars for Docs: How industry dollars reach your doctors. Propublica. Updated 24 Sept 2013. Available: http://projects.propublica.org/docdollars/. Accessed Dec 13, 2013.

13 The Center For Responsive Politics. Influence & lobbying - lobbying database. Updated 31 Oct 2011. Available: http://www.opensecrets.org/lobby/. Accessed Dec 11, 2011.

14 Himmelstein DU, Thorne D, Warren E, et al. Medical bankruptcy in the United States, 2007: results of a national study. Am J Med. 2009 Aug;122(8):741-6.

15 Barnard ND. Trends in food availability, 1909-2007. Am J Clin Nutr. 2010;91:1530S-1536S.

16 Drewnowski A, Darmon N. The economics of obesity: dietary energy density and energy cost. Am J Clin Nutr. 2005 Jul;82(1 Suppl):265S-273S.

17 Environmental Working Group, "Farm Subsidy Database,". Available: http://farm.ewg.org/ (updated June 2011). Accessed Dec 17, 2011.

18 Institute for Agriculture and Trade Policy. Below-cost feed crops: an indirect subsidy for industrial animal factories. IATP. June 2006. Available: http://www.nffc.net/Learn/Reports/BelowCost6_06.pdf. Accessed Dec 17, 2011.

19 Ralph Chite and Dennis Shields, "Dairy Policy and the 2008 Farm Bill," Congressional Research Service RL34036 (Jan. 22, 2009).

20 United States Department of Agriculture. Dairy Price Support Program. Available: http://georgewbush-whitehouse.archives.gov/omb/expectmore/summary/10002436.2006.html. Accessed Dec 17, 2011.

21 Environmental Working Group, "Farm Subsidy Database,". Available: http://farm.ewg.org/ (updated June 2011). Accessed Dec 17, 2011.

22 United States Department of Agriculture. Environmental Quality Incentives Program. Available: http://www.nrcs.usda.gov/programs/eqip/. Accessed Dec 17, 2011.

23 Dennis Shields, "Federal Crop Insurance: Background and Issues," Congressional Research Service R40532 (Dec. 13, 2010).

24 The Center For Responsive Politics. Influence & lobbying - lobbying database. Updated 31 Oct 2011. Available: http://www.opensecrets.org/lobby/. Accessed Dec 17, 2011.

25 Centers for Disease Control and Prevention. CDC's mission and vision. Available: http://www.cdc.gov/about/organization/cio.htm. Accessed Dec 17, 2011.

26 United States Department of Agriculture. Mission statement. Available: http://www.usda.gov/wps/portal/usda/usdahome?navid=MISSION_STATEMENT. Accessed Dec 17, 2011.

Chapter 9 - A Healthful New Menu

1 He FJ, MacGregor GA. Beneficial effects of potassium on human health. Physiol Plant. 2008 Aug;133(4):725-35.

2 Nikolic M, Nikic D, Petrovic B. Fruit and vegetable intake and the risk for developing coronary heart disease. Cent Eur J Public Health. 2008 Mar;16(1):17-20.

3 Vrecer M, Turk S, et al. Use of statins in primary and secondary prevention of coronary heart disease and ischemic stroke. Meta-analysis of randomized trials. Int J Clin Pharmacol Ther. 2003 Dec;41(12):567-77.

4 Zafra-Stone S, Yasmin T, et al. Berry anthocyanins as novel antioxidants in human health and disease prevention. Mol Nutr Food Res. 2007 Jun; 51(6):675-83.

5 Camacho L, Sierra C, et al. Nutritional changes caused by the germination of legumes commonly eaten in Chile. Arch Latinoam Nutr. 1992 Sep;42 (3):283-90.

6 Trinidad TP, Mallillin AC, et al. The potential health benefits of legumes as a good source of dietary fibre. Br J Nutr. 2010 Feb;103(4):569-74.

7 Messina MJ. Legumes and soybeans: overview of their nutritional profiles and health effects. Am J Clin Nutr. 1999 Sept;70(3):439S-450S.

8 Sarkar FH, Li Y. Soy isoflavones and cancer prevention. Cancer Invest. 2003;21(5):744-57.

9 Wu AH, Yu MC, et al. Epidemiology of soy exposures and breast cancer risk. Br J Canc. 2008 Jan 15;98(1):9-14.

10 Yang G, Shu XO, et al. Prospective cohort study of soy food intake and colorectal cancer risk in women. Am J Clin Nutr. 2009 Feb;89(2):577-83.

11 Jonnalaggada SS, Harnack L, et al. Putting the Whole Grain Puzzle Together: Health Benefits Associated with Whole Grains—Summary of American Society for Nutrition 2010 Satellite Symposium. J Nutr. 2011 May;141(5): 1011S–1022S.

12 Simopoulos AP. Essential fatty acids in health and chronic disease. Am J Clin Nutr. 1999 Sep;70(3 Suppl):560S-569S.

13 Lehraiki A, Attoumbré J, Bienaimé C, et al. Extraction of lignans from flaxseed and evaluation of their biological effects on breast cancer MCF-7 and MDA-MB-231 cell lines. J Med Food. 2010 Aug;13(4):834-41.

14 Jenab M, Thompson LU. The influence of flaxseed and lignans on colon carcinogenesis and beta-glucuronidase activity. Carcinogenesis. 1996 Jun; 17(6):1343-8.

1 Denke MA. Dietary fats, fatty acids, and their effects on lipoproteins. Curr Atheroscler Rep. 2006 Nov;8(6):466-71.

2 Merchant AT, Kelemen LE, et al. Interrelation of saturated fat, trans fat, alcohol intake, and subclinical atherosclerosis. Am J Clin Nutr. 2008 Jan; 87(1):168-174.

3 Kalmijn S. Fatty acid intake and the risk of dementia and cognitive decline: a review of clinical and epidemiological studies. J Nutr Health Aging. 2000;4(4):202-7.

4 Hu FB, van Dam RM, Liu S. Diet and risk of Type II diabetes: the role of types of fat and carbohydrate. Diabetologia. 2001 Jul;44(7):805-17. Review.

5 Behrman EJ, Gopalan V. Cholesterol and plants. J Chem Edu. 2005;82: 1791-1793.

6 Hu FB. Plant-based foods and prevention of cardiovascular disease: an overview. Am J Clin Nutr. 2003 Sept;78(3):544S-551S.

7 Vogel RA, Corretti MC, Plotnick GD. The postprandial effect of components of the Mediterranean diet on endothelial function. 2000;36:1455-1460.

8 Tokudome S, Nagaya T, et al. Japanese versus Mediterranean diets and cancer. Asian Pac J Canc Prev. 2000;1:61-66.

9 Simopoulos AP. The importance of the omega-6/omega-3 fatty acid ratio in cardiovascular disease and other chronic diseases. Exp Biol Med (Maywood). 2008 Jun;233(6):674-88.

10 Luopajärvi K, Savilahti E, et al. Enhanced levels of cow's milk antibodies in infancy in children who develop type 1 diabetes later in childhood. Pediatr Diabetes. 2008 Oct;9(5):434-41.

11 Knip M, Suvi VM, et al. Dietary Intervention in Infancy and Later Signs of Beta-Cell Autoimmunity. N Engl J Med. 2010 Nov;363:1900-1908.

12 Chen Z, Hu J, et al. Inhibition of hepatocellular carcinoma development in hepatitis B virus transfected mice by low dietary casein. Hepatology. 1997 Nov;26(5):1351-4.

13 Madhavan TV, Gopalan C. The effect of dietary protein on carcinogenesis of aflatoxin. Arch Pathol. 1968 Feb;85(2):133-7.

14 van der Pols JC, Bain C, et al. Childhood dairy intake and adult cancer risk: 65-y follow-up of the Boyd Orr cohort. Am J Clin Nutr. 2007 Dec; 86(6):1722-9.

15 Gonzalez CA, Riboli E. Diet and cancer prevention: Contributions from the European Prospective Investigation into Cancer and Nutrition (EPIC) study. 2010 Sept;46(14):2555-2562.

16 Larsson SC, Orsini N, Wolk A. Milk, milk products and lactose intake and ovarian cancer risk: A meta-analysis of epidemiological studies. Int J Cancer. 2005 Jul;118:431-441.

17 Danby FW. Acne, dairy and cancer. Dermatoendocrinol. 2009 Jan-Feb;1(1): 12–16.

18 Bulletin of the International Dairy Federation 446/2010. The World Dairy Situation 2010. Belgium.

19 Dhanwal DK, Cooper C, et al. Geographic Variation in Osteoporotic Hip Fracture Incidence: The Growing Importance of Asian Influences in Coming Decades. J Osteoporos. 2010;2010:757102.

20 Heaney RP, Layman DK. Amount and type of protein influences bone health. Am J Clin Nutr. 2008 May;87(5):1567S-1570S. Review.

21 Calvo MS, Uribarri J. Public health impact of dietary phosphorus excess on bone and cardiovascular health in the general population. Am J Clin Nutr. 2013 Jul;98(1):6-15.

22 Karp H, Ekholm P, Kemi V, et al. Differences among total and in vitro digestible phosphorus content of meat and milk products. J Ren Nutr. 2012 May;22(3):344-9.

23 Murphy CG, O'Flanagan S, Keogh P, Kenny P. Subtrochanteric stress fractures in patients on oral bisphosphonate therapy: an emerging problem. Acta Orthop Belg. 2011 Oct;77(5):632-7.

24 Newman, D. Bisphosphonates for Fracture Prevention in Post-Menopausal Women Without Prior Fractures. theNNT. 2011 May 16. Available: http://www.thennt.com/nnt/bisphosphonates-for-fracture-prevention-in-post-menopausal-women-without-prior-fractures/. Accessed Mar 21, 2014.

25 Newman, D. Bisphosphonates for Fracture Prevention in Post-Menopausal Women With Prior Fractures or With Very Low Bone Density. Available: http://www.thennt.com/nnt/bisphosphonates-for-fracture-prevention-in-post-menopausal-women-with-prior-fractures-or-very-low-bone-density/. Accessed Mar 21, 2014.

26 Hertzler SR, Huynh BCL, Savaiano DA. How much lactose is low lactose? J Am Dietetic Asso. 1996;96:243-246.

27 Djoussé L, Gaziano JM. Egg consumption in relation to cardiovascular disease and mortality: the Physicians' Health Study. Am J Clin Nutr. 2008 Apr;87(4):964-9.

28 Djoussé L, Gaziano JM, et al. Egg consumption and risk of type 2 diabetes in men and women. Diabetes Care. 2009 Feb;32(2):295-300.

29 Richman EL, Stampfer MJ, et al. Intakes of meat, fish, poultry, and eggs and risk of prostate cancer progression. Am J Clin Nutr. 2010 Mar; 91(3):712-721.

30 Richman EL, Kenfield SA, et al. Egg, red meat, and poultry intake and risk of lethal prostate cancer in the prostate specific antigen-era: incidence and survival. Cancer Prev Res. Published ahead of print September 19, 2011; DOI:10.1158/1940-6207.CAPR-11-0354.

31 Wells HF, Buzby JC. Dietary Assessment of Major Trends in U.S. Food Consumption, 1970-2005. Economic Information Bulletin No. (EIB-33) 27 pp. March 2008. Available: http://www.ers.usda.gov/Publications/EIB33/.

32 Hu FB. Are refined carbohydrates worse than saturated fat? Am J Clin Nutr. 2010 June; 91(6):1541-1542.

33 Akbaraly TN, Brunner EJ, et al. Dietary pattern and depressive symptoms in middle age. Br J Psychiatry. 2009 Nov;195(5):408-13.

34 Centers for Disease Control. Sodium intake among adults - United States, 2005-2006. MMWR Morb Mortal Wkly Rep. 2010 Jun 25;59(24):746-9.

35 Smith-Spangler CM, Juusola JL, et al. Population strategies to decrease sodium intake and the burden of cardiovascular disease: a cost-effectiveness analysis. Ann Intern Med. 2010 Apr 20;152(8):481-7,W170-3.

36 Strazzullo P, D'Elia L, et al. Salt intake, stroke, and cardiovascular disease: meta-analysis of prospective studies. BMJ. 2009;339:b4567.

37 Ni Mhurchu C, Capelin C, et al. Sodium content of processed foods in the United Kingdom: analysis of 44,000 foods purchased by 21,000 households. Am J Clin Nutr. 2011 Mar;93(3):594-600.

38 Bamford J, Dennis M, et al. The frequency, causes and timing of death within 30 days of a first stroke: the Oxfordshire Community Stroke Project. J Neurol Neurosurg Psychiatry. 1990 October;53(10):824-829.

39 Suzuki K, Izumi M, et al. Blood pressure and total cholesterol level are critical risks especially for hemorrhagic stroke in Akita, Japan. Cerebrovasc Dis. 2011;31(1):100-6.

40 Truelsen T, Begg S, Mathers C. The global burden of cerebrovascular disease. World Health Organization. 2000. Available: http://www.who.int/healthinfo/statistics/bod_cerebrovasculardiseasestroke.pdf.

41 Japanese Ministry of Health, Labour, and Welfare. Outline of Results from 2007 National Health and Nutrition Survey. Available: www.mhlw.go.jp/english/wp/wp-hw3/dl/2-064_065.pdf.

Chapter 11 - The Gluten-Free Diet Craze

1 Wong, V. Gluten-Free Shoppers Like Snacks Too. Bloomberg Businessweek. 2013 May 16.

2 Hischenhuber C, Crevel R, Jarry B, et al. Review article: safe amounts of gluten for patients with wheat allergy or coeliac disease. Aliment Pharmacol Ther. 2006 Mar 1;23(5):559-75. Review.

3 Gujral N, Freeman HJ, Thomson AB. Celiac disease: prevalence, diagnosis, pathogenesis and treatment. World J Gastroenterol. 2012 Nov 14;18(42): 6036-59.

4 Sapone A, Bai JC, Ciacci C, et al. Spectrum of gluten-related disorders: consensus on new nomenclature and classification. BMC Med. 2012 Feb 7; 10:13. Review.

5 Garsed K, Scott BB. Can oats be taken in a gluten-free diet? A systematic review. Scand J Gastroenterol. 2007 Feb;42(2):171-8. Review.

6 Rubio-Tapia A, Hill ID, Kelly CP, et al. ACG clinical guidelines: diagnosis and management of celiac disease. Am J Gastroenterol. 2013 May;108(5):656-76. Epub 2013 Apr 23.

7 Kaukinen K, Collin P, Mäki M. Latent coeliac disease or coeliac disease beyond villous atrophy? Gut. 2007 Oct;56(10):1339-40.

8 Kneepkens CM, von Blomberg BM. Clinical practice : Coeliac disease. Eur J Pediatr. 2012 Jul;171(7):1011-21.

9 Gujral N, Freeman HJ, Thomson AB. Celiac disease: prevalence, diagnosis, pathogenesis and treatment. World J Gastroenterol. 2012 Nov 14;18 (42):6036-59.

10 Criado PR, Criado RF, Aoki V, et al. Dermatitis herpetiformis: relevance of the physical examination to diagnosis suspicion. Can Fam Physician. 2012 Aug;58(8):843-7.

11 Hadjivassiliou M, Sanders DS, Woodroofe N, et al. Gluten ataxia. Cerebellum. 2008;7(3):494-8. Review.

12 Hadjivassiliou M, Grünewald R, Sharrack B, et al. Gluten ataxia in perspective: epidemiology, genetic susceptibility and clinical characteristics. Brain. 2003 Mar;126(Pt 3):685-91.

13 Muzaimi MB, Thomas J, Palmer-Smith S, et al. Population based study of late onset cerebellar ataxia in southeast Wales. J Neurol Neurosurg Psychiatry. 2004 Aug;75(8):1129-34.

14 Pietzak M. Celiac disease, wheat allergy, and gluten sensitivity: when gluten free is not a fad. JPEN J Parenter Enteral Nutr. 2012 Jan;36(1 Suppl): 68S-75S. Review.

15 Hagemeyer O, Bünger J, van Kampen V, et al. Respiratory allergy in apprentice bakers: do occupational allergies follow the allergic march? Adv Exp Med Biol. 2013;788:313-20.

16 Siles RI, Hsieh FH. Allergy blood testing: A practical guide for clinicians. Cleve Clin J Med. 2011 Sep;78(9):585-92. Review.

17 Morita E, Chinuki Y, Takahashi H, et al. Prevalence of wheat allergy in Japanese adults. Allergol Int. 2012 Mar;61(1):101-5.

18 Brown AC. Gluten sensitivity: problems of an emerging condition separate from celiac disease. Expert Rev Gastroenterol Hepatol. 2012 Feb;6(1): 43-55. Review.

19 Lundin KE, Alaedini A. Non-celiac gluten sensitivity. Gastrointest Endosc Clin N Am. 2012 Oct;22(4):723-34. Review.

20 Jackson JR, Eaton WW, Cascella NG, et al. Neurologic and psychiatric manifestations of celiac disease and gluten sensitivity. Psychiatr Q. 2012 Mar;83(1): 91-102. Review.

21 White MC. Why We're Wasting Billions On Gluten-Free Food. Time Magazine. 2013 Mar 13.

22 De Palma G, Nadal I, Collado MC, Sanz Y. Effects of a gluten-free diet on gut microbiota and immune function in healthy adult human subjects. Br J Nutr. 2009 Oct;102(8):1154-60.

Chapter 13 - A Nation of Addicts

1 American Cancer Society. *Cancer Facts and Figures 2011*. Atlanta: American Cancer Society; 2011.

2 Hernandez L, Hoebel BG. Food reward and cocaine increase extracellular dopamine in the nucleus accumbens as measured by microdialysis. Life Sci. 1988;42(18):1705-12.

3 Merriam-Webster, Inc. Definition of Addiction. Available: http://www.merriam-webster.com/dictionary/addiction. Accessed October 22, 2011.

4 Lisle DJ, Goldhamer A. The Pleasure Trap. Summertown, TN: Healthy Living Publications. 2003.

5   Arias-Carrión O, Pöppel E. Dopamine, learning, and reward-seeking behavior. Act Neurobiol Exp. 2007;67(4):481–488.

6   Volkow ND, Wang GJ, Fowler JS, et al. Addiction: decreased reward sensitivity and increased expectation sensitivity conspire to overwhelm the brain's control circuit. Bioessays. 2010 Sep;32(9):748-755. Review.

7   Avena NM, Rada P, Hoebel BG. Sugar and Fat Bingeing Have Notable Differences in Addictive-like Behavior. J Nutr. 2009 March;139(3):623–628.

8   Cooper SJ, Al-Naser HA. Dopaminergic control of food choice: contrasting effects of SKF 38393 and quinpirole on high-palatability food preference in the rat. Neuropharmacology. 2006 Jun;50(8):953-63.

9   Cocores JA, Gold MS. The Salted Food Addiction Hypothesis may explain overeating and the obesity epidemic. Med Hypotheses. 2009 Dec; 73(6):892-9.

10 Lutter M, Nestler EJ. Homeostatic and Hedonic Signals Interact in the Regulation of Food Intake. J Nutr. 2009 March;139(3):629–632.

11 Leibowitz, SF. Overconsumption of dietary fat and alcohol: Mechanisms involving lipids and hypothalamic peptides. Physiol Behav. 2007 Aug 15; 91(5):513-521.

12 Chang GQ, Karatayev O, Ahsan R, et al. Effect of ethanol on hypothalamic opioid peptides, enkephalin, and dynorphin: relationship with circulating triglycerides. Alcohol Clin Exp Res. 2007 Feb;31(2):249-59.

13 Leibowitz SF. Regulation and effects of hypothalamic galanin: relation to dietary fat, alcohol ingestion, circulating lipids and energy homeostasis. Neuropeptides. 2005;39:327–332.

14 Avena NM, Rada P, Hoebel BG. Evidence for sugar addiction: Behavioral and neurochemical effects of intermittent, excessive sugar intake. Neurosci Biobehav Rev. 2008;32(1):20-39.

15 Avena NM, Bocarsly ME, Rada P, et al. After daily bingeing on a sucrose solution, food deprivation induces anxiety and accumbens dopamine/acetylcholine imbalance. Physiol Behav. 2008 Jun 9;94(3):309-15.

16 Teschemacher H, Koch G, Brantl V. Milk protein-derived opioid receptor ligands. Biopolymers. 1997;43(2):99-117.

17 Kost NV, Sokolov OY, Kurasova OB, et al. Beta-casomorphins-7 in infants on different type of feeding and different levels of psychomotor development. Peptides. 2009 Oct;30(10):1854-60.

18 Kaminski S, Cieslinska A, Kostyra E. Polymorphism of bovine beta-casein and its potential effect on human health. J Apple Genet. 2007;48(3):189-98

19 Parylak SL, Koob GF, Zorrilla EP. The dark side of food addiction. Physiol Behav. 2011 Jul 25;104(1):149-56.

20 Jamel HA, Sheiham A, Cowell CR, Watt RG. Taste preference for sweetness in urban and rural populations in Iraq. J Dent Res. 1996 Nov; 75(11):1879-84.

21 Zhang XJ, Zhou LH, Ban X, et al. Decreased expression of CD36 in circumvallate taste buds of high-fat diet induced obese rats. Acta Histochem. 2011 Oct;113(6):663-7.

22 Bertino M, Beauchamp GK, Engelman K. Long-term reduction in dietary sodium alters the taste of salt. Am J Clin Nutr. 1982 Dec;36(6):1134-44.

1   Campbell TC, Campbell II TM. The China Study. Dallas, TX: Benbella Books, Inc. 2006.

2   Soloviev M, Barry R, et al. Combinatorial peptidomics: a generic approach for protein expression profiling. J Nanobiotechnology. 2003 Jul 3;1(1):4.

3   Wahl C, Hess B. [Kidney calculi--is nutrition a trigger or treatment?]. Ther Umsch. 2000 Mar;57(3):138-45. Review.

4   Halbesma N, Bakker S, et al. High Protein Intake Associates with Cardiovascular Events but not with Loss of Renal Function. J Am Soc Nephrol. 2009 August;20(8):1797–1804.

5   Joint FAO/WHO/UNU Expert Consultation. Protein and Amino Acid Requirements in Human Nutrition. WHO Library Cataloguing-in-Publication Data. 2002;8.3:149-150.

6   Fulgoni VL 3rd. Current protein intake in America: analysis of the National Health and Nutrition Examination Survey, 2003-2004. Am J Clin Nutr. 2008 May;87(5):1554S-1557S.

7   Hardage M. Nutritional studies of vegetarians. Journal of the American Dietetic Association. 1966;48:25.

8   Tarnopolsky MA, Atkinson SA, MacDougall JD, et al. Evaluation of protein requirements for trained strength athletes. J Appl Physiol. 1992 Nov; 73(5):1986-95.

9   Phillips SM, Moore DR, Tang JE. A critical examination of dietary protein requirements, benefits, and excesses in athletes. Int J Sport Nutr Exerc Metab. 2007 Aug;17 Suppl:S58-76. Review.

10 Kreider RB, Campbell B. Protein for exercise and recovery. Phys Sportsmed. 2009 Jun;37(2):13-21. Review.

11 Selden MA, Helzberg JH, Waeckerle JF. Early cardiovascular mortality in professional football players: fact or fiction? Am J Med. 2009 Sep;122(9): 811-4. Review.

12 Samaras TT, Storms LH, Elrick H. Longevity, mortality and body weight. Ageing Res Rev. 2002 Sep;1(4):673-91. Review.

13 National Institutes For Health. Congenital Protein C and S deficiency. Medline Plus. Available: http://www.nlm.nih.gov/medlineplus/ency/article/000559.htm. Accessed Nov 10, 2011.

14 Kotler DP. Cachexia. Ann Int Med. 2000 Oct 17;133(8):622-634.

15 Kumar NB, Kazi A, Smith T, et al. Cancer Cachexia: Traditional Therapies and Novel Molecular Mechanism-Based Approaches to Treatment. Current Treatment Options in Oncology. 2010;11(3-4):107-117.

16 Jahoor F, Badaloo A, Reid M, et al. Protein metabolism in severe childhood malnutrition. Ann Trop Paediatr. 2008 Jun;28(2):87-101. Review.

17 Young VR. Adult Amino acid requirements: The case for a major revision in current recommendations. Jour of Nutrition. 1994;124:1517S-1523S.

18 McDougall J. Plant foods have a complete amino acid composition. Circulation. 2002 Jun 25;105(25):e197; author reply e197.

19 Lovelock JE, Porterfield BM. Blood clotting; the function of electrolytes and of calcium. Biochem J. 1952 Jan;50(3):415-20.

20 Cartwright EJ, Schuh K, Neyses L. Calcium transport in cardiovascular health and disease—the sarcolemmal calcium pump enters the stage. J Mol Cell Cardiol. 2005 Sep;39(3):403-6. Review.

21 Food and Nutrition Board, Institute of Medicine. Calcium. Dietary Reference Intakes: Calcium, Phosphorus, Magnesium, Vitamin D, and Fluoride. Washington, D.C.: National Academy Press; 1997:71-145.

22 Committee to Review Dietary Reference Intakes for Vitamin D and Calcium, Institute of Medicine. "Front Matter." Dietary Reference Intakes for Calcium and Vitamin D. Washington, DC: The National Academies Press, 2011.

23 Hunt CD, Johnson LK. Calcium requirements: new estimations for men and women by cross-sectional statistical analyses of calcium balance data from metabolic studies. Am J Clin Nutr. 2007 Oct;86(4):1054-63.

24 Weaver CM, Proulx WR, Heaney RP. Choices for achieving adequate dietary calcium with a vegetarian diet. Am J Clin Nutr 1999;70:543S-8S.

25 Massey LK, Whiting SJ. Caffeine, urinary calcium, calcium metabolism, and bone. J Nutr 1993;123:1611-4.

26 Sax L. The institute of medicine's "dietary reference intake" for phosphorus: a critical perspective. Am Coll Nutr. 2001 Aug;20(4):271-8. Review.

27 Heaney RP, Weaver CM, et al. Absorbability of Calcium from Brassica Vegetables: Broccoli, Bok Choy, and Kale. J Food Sci. 1993 Nov;58(6):1378-1380.

28 Grusak MA, Abrams SA. Bioavailability of Calcium from Common Vegetables Assessed in Teenagers. HotScience. 1996 Aug;31(4)644.

29 Heaney RP, Weaver CM, Recker RR. Calcium absorbability from spinach. Am J Clin Nutr. 1988 Apr;47(4):707-9.

30 Fraser GE. Vegetarian diets: what do we know of their effects on common chronic diseases? Am J Clin Nutr. 2009 May; 89(5):1607S–1612S.

31 Willcox DC, Willcox BJ, Todoriki H, et al. The Okinawan diet: health implications of a low-calorie, nutrient-dense, antioxidant-rich dietary pattern low in glycemic load. J Am Coll Nutr. 2009 Aug;28 Suppl:500S-516S. Review.

32 Barnard ND, Gloede L, Cohen J, et al. A low-fat vegan diet elicits greater macronutrient changes, but is comparable in adherence and acceptability, compared with a more conventional diabetes diet among individuals with type 2 diabetes. J Am Diet Assoc. 2009 Feb;109(2):263-72.

33 Barnard ND, Scialli AR, et al. Acceptability of a low-fat vegan diet compares favorably to a step II diet in a randomized, controlled trial. J Cardiopulm Rehabil. 2004 Jul-Aug;24(4):229-35.

34 Stanger J. Vegan from the inside: why people love plant-based diets. 2011. Available: http://perfectformuladiet.com/wp-content/uploads/2011/02/Vegan-from-the-Inside-rept.pdf. Accessed Nov 27, 2011.

35 Weijs PJ, Kool LM, et al. High beverage sugar as well as high animal protein intake at infancy may increase overweight risk at 8 years: a prospective longitudinal pilot study. Nutr J. 2011 Sep 23;10:95.

36 Matthews VL, Wien M, Sabaté J. The risk of child and adolescent overweight is related to types of food consumed. Nutr J. 2011 Jun 24;10:71.

37 Frank GC, Farris RP, et al. Dietary trends of 10- and 13-year-old children in a bi-racial community—the Bogalusa Heart Study. Prev Med. 1985 Jan;14(1):123-39.

38 Fuemmeler BF, Pendzich MK, Tercyak KP. Weight, dietary behavior, and physical activity in childhood and adolescence: implications for adult cancer risk. Obes Facts. 2009;2(3):179-86. Epub 2009 Jun 4. Review.

39 Sabaté J, Wien M. Vegetarian diets and childhood obesity prevention. Am J Clin Nutr. 2010 May;91(5):1525S-1529S.

40 Furhman J. Spotlight on children's health issues. Available: http://www.drfuhrman.com/children/default.aspx. Accessed Nov 27, 2011.

Chapter 15 - Move It or Lose It—The Benefits of Exercising

1 BeFit Enterprises. "Jack LaLanne - The King of Fitness." Available: http://www.jacklalanne.com/. Accessed Dec 29, 2011.

2 Woodcock J, Franco OH, Orsini N, et al. Non-vigorous physical activity and all-cause mortality: systematic review and meta-analysis of cohort studies. Int J Epidemiol. 2011 Feb;40(1):121-38.

3 Warburton DE, Nicol CW, Bredin SS. Health benefits of physical activity: the evidence. CMAJ. 2006 Mar 14;174(6):801-9.

4 Ludlow AT, Roth SM. Physical Activity and Telomere Biology: Exploring the Link with Aging-Related Disease Prevention. J Aging Res. 2011;2011:790378.

5 Ludlow AT, Zimmerman JB, Witkowski S, et al. Relationship between physical activity level, telomere length, and telomerase activity. Med Sci Sports Exerc. 2008 Oct;40(10):1764-71.

6 Garber CE, Blissmer B, Deschenes MR, et al. American College of Sports Medicine position stand. Quantity and quality of exercise for developing and maintaining cardiorespiratory, musculoskeletal, and neuromotor fitness in apparently healthy adults: guidance for prescribing exercise. Med Sci Sports Exerc. 2011 Jul;43(7):1334-59.

7 McHugh MP, Cosgrave CH. To stretch or not to stretch: the role of stretching in injury prevention and performance. Scand J Med Sci Sports. 2010 Apr;20(2):169-81.

8 Roberts JM, Wilson K. Effect of stretching duration on active and passive range of motion in the lower extremity. Br J Sports Med. 1999 Aug;33(4):259-63.

9 Miller MG, Herniman JJ, Ricard MD, et al. The effects of a 6-week plyometric training program on agility. J of Spo Sci & Med. 2006;(5):459-465.

10 Li Y, Devault CN, Van Oteghen S. Effects of extended Tai Chi intervention on balance and selected motor functions of the elderly. Am J Chin Med. 2007;35(3):383-91.

11 Jahnke R, Larkey L, Rogers C, et al. A comprehensive review of health benefits of qigong and tai chi. Am J Health Promot. 2010 Jul-Aug;24(6): e1-e25. Review.

12 Rogers CE, Larkey LK, Keller C. A review of clinical trials of tai chi and qigong in older adults. West J Nurs Res. 2009 Mar;31(2):245-79. Review.

13 Ratel S. High-intensity and resistance training and elite young athletes. Med Sport Sci. 2011;56:84-96. Epub 2010 Dec 21. Review.

14 Phillips SM. Resistance exercise: good for more than just Grandma and Grandpa's muscles. Appl Physiol Nutr Metab. 2007 Dec;32(6): 1198-205. Review.

15 Balakrishnan VS, Rao M, Menon V, et al. Resistance training increases muscle mitochondrial biogenesis in patients with chronic kidney disease. Clin J Am Soc Nephrol. 2010 Jun;5(6):996-1002.

16 Guadalupe-Grau A, Fuentes T, Guerra B, Calbet JA. Exercise and bone mass in adults. Sports Med. 2009;39(6):439-68. Review.

17 Weil, R. Aerobic Exercise: How much do I need to gain all these benefits? Available: http://www.emedicinehealth.com/aerobic_exercise/. Accessed Jan 9, 2012.

18 Camarda SR, Tebexreni AS, Páfaro CN, et al. Comparison of maximal heart rate using the prediction equations proposed by Karvonen and Tanaka. Arq Bras Cardiol. 2008 Nov;91(5):311-4.

19 Mersy DJ. Health benefits of aerobic exercise. Postgrad Med. 1991 Jul;90(1):103-7,110-2.

20 Reid KJ, Baron KG, Lu B, et al. Aerobic exercise improves self-reported sleep and quality of life in older adults with insomnia. Sleep Med. 2010 Oct;11(9):934-40.

Chapter 16 - Supplement Wisely

1 Cloud J. Nutrition in a pill? Time Magazine. 2011 Sep 12.

2 Redberg RF. Vitamin supplements: More cost than value. Arch Intern Med. 2011 Oct 10;171(18):1634-1635.

3 Gahche J, Bailey R, Burt V, et al. Dietary supplement use among U.S. adults has increased since NHANES III (1988-1994). NCHS Data Brief. 2011 Apr;(61):1-8.

4 Mursu J, Robien K, Harnack LJ, et al. Dietary Supplements and Mortality Rate in Older Women. Arch Intern Med. 2011 Oct 10;171(18):1625-1633.

5 Larsson SC, Akesson A, Bergkvist L, et al. Multivitamin use and breast cancer incidence in a prospective cohort of Swedish women. Am J Clin Nutr. 2010 May;91(5):1268-72.

6 Morimoto LM, White E, Chen Z, et al. Obesity, body size, and risk of postmenopausal breast cancer: the Women's Health Initiative (United States). Cancer Causes Control. 2002 Oct;13(8):741-51.

7 Giovannucci E, Chan AT. Role of vitamin and mineral supplementation and aspirin use in cancer survivors. J Clin Oncol. 2010 Sep 10;28(26):4081-5.

8 Lawson KA, Wright ME, Subar A, et al. Multivitamin use and risk of prostate cancer in the National Institutes of Health-AARP Diet and Health Study. J Natl Cancer Inst. 2007 May 16;99(10):754-64.

9 Woodside JV, McCall D, McGartland C, et al. Micronutrients: dietary intake v. supplement use. Proc Nutr Soc. 2005 Nov;64(4):543-53. Review.

10 Marra MV, Wellman NS. Multivitamin-mineral supplements in the Older Americans Act Nutrition Program: not a one-size-fits-all quick fix. Am J Public Health. 2008 Jul;98(7):1171-6.

11 Lee IM, Cook NR, Gaziano JM, et al. Vitamin E in the primary prevention of cardiovascular disease and cancer: the Women's Health Study: a randomized controlled trial. JAMA. 2005 Jul 6;294(1):56-65.

12 Liu S, Lee IM, Song Y, et al. Vitamin E and risk of type 2 diabetes in the women's health study randomized controlled trial. Diabetes. 2006 Oct;55 (10):2856-62.

13 Sesso HD, Buring JE, Christen WG, Kurth T, Belanger C, MacFadyen J, et al. Vitamins E and C in the prevention of cardiovascular disease in men: the Physicians' Health Study II randomized controlled trial. JAMA 2008; 300:2123-33.

14 Klein EA, Thompson IM Jr, Tangen CM, et al. Vitamin E and the risk of prostate cancer: the Selenium and Vitamin E Cancer Prevention Trial (SELECT). JAMA. 2011 Oct 12;306(14):1549-56.

15 Dotan Y, Lichtenberg D, Pinchuk I. No evidence supports vitamin E indiscriminate supplementation. Biofactors. 2009 Nov-Dec;35(6):469-73. Review.

16 Institute of Medicine. Food and Nutrition Board. Dietary Reference Intakes: Vitamin C, Vitamin E, Selenium, and Carotenoids. Washington, DC: National Academy Press, 2000.

17 Hinds TS, West WL, Knight EM. Carotenoids and retinoids: A review of research, clinical, and public health applications. J Clin Pharmacol 1997; 37:551-8.

18 Albanes D, Heinonen OP, Taylor PR, et al. Alpha-tocopherol and beta-carotene supplement and lung cancer incidence in the alpha-tocopherol, beta-carotene cancer prevention study: Effects of base-line characteristics and study compliance. J Natl Cancer Inst 1996;88:1560-70.

19 Bendich A, Langseth L. Safety of vitamin A. Am J Clin Nutr. 1989 Feb;49(2): 358-371. Review.

20 Feskanich D, Singh V, Willett WC, et al. Vitamin A intake and hip fractures among postmenopausal women. JAMA. 2002 Jan 2;287(1):47-54.

21 Johansson S, Melhus H. Vitamin A antagonizes calcium response to vitamin D in man. J Bone Miner Res. 2001 Oct;16(10):1899-905.

22 Institute of Medicine. Food and Nutrition Board. Dietary Reference Intakes for Vitamin A, Vitamin K, Arsenic, Boron, Chromium, Copper, Iodine, Iron, Manganese, Molybdenum, Nickel, Silicon, Vanadium, and Zinc. National Academy Press, Washington, DC, 2001.

23 Pintó X, Vilaseca MA, Balcells S, et al. A folate-rich diet is as effective as folic acid from supplements in decreasing plasma homocysteine concentrations. Int J Med Sci. 2005;2(2):58-63.

24 Shaw GM, Schaffer D, Velie EM, et al. Periconceptional vitamin use, dietary folate, and the occurrence of neural tube defects. Epidemiology 1995; 6:219-26.

25 Miller ER 3rd, Juraschek S, Pastor-Barriuso R, et al. Meta-analysis of folic acid supplementation trials on risk of cardiovascular disease and risk interaction with baseline homocysteine levels. Am J Cardiol. 2010 Aug 15;106(4):517-27.

26 Cui R, Iso H, Date C, et al. Dietary folate and vitamin b6 and B12 intake in relation to mortality from cardiovascular diseases: Japan collaborative cohort study. Stroke. 2010 Jun;41(6):1285-9.

27 Fife J, Raniga S, Hider PN, Frizelle FA. Folic acid supplementation and colorectal cancer risk: a meta-analysis. Colorectal Dis. 2011 Feb;13(2):132-7.

28 Figueiredo JC, Grau MV, Haile RW, et al. Folic acid and risk of prostate cancer: results from a randomized clinical trial. J Natl Cancer Inst. 2009 Mar 18;101(6):432-5.

29 Kim YI. Does a high folate intake increase the risk of breast cancer? Nutr Rev. 2006 Oct;64(10 Pt 1):468-475. Review.

30 Iyer R, Tomar SK. Folate: a functional food constituent. J Food Sci. 2009 Nov-Dec;74(9):R114-22. Review.

31 Calder PC, Yaqoob P. Omega-3 polyunsaturated fatty acids and human health outcomes. Biofactors. 2009 May-Jun;35(3):266-72. Review.

32 Bushkin-Bedient S, Carpenter DO. Benefits versus risks associated with consumption of fish and other seafood. Rev Environ Health. 2010 Jul-Sep;25(3): 161-191. Review.

33 Brouwer IA, Katan MB, Zock PL. Dietary alpha-linolenic acid is associated with reduced risk of fatal coronary heart disease, but increased prostate cancer risk: a meta-analysis. J Nutr. 2004 Apr;134(4):919-22.

34 Demark-Wahnefried W, Polascik TJ, George SL, et al. Flaxseed supplementation (not dietary fat restriction) reduces prostate cancer proliferation rates in men presurgery. Cancer Epidemiol Biomarkers Prev. 2008 Dec; 17(12):3577-87.

35 Chen J, Stavro PM, Thompson LU. Dietary flaxseed inhibits human breast cancer growth and metastasis and downregulates expression of insulin-like growth factor and epidermal growth factor receptor. Nutr Cancer. 2002; 43(2):187-92.

36 Lowcock EC, Cotterchio M, Boucher BA. Consumption of flaxseed, a rich source of lignans, is associated with reduced breast cancer risk. Cancer Causes Control. 2013 Apr;24(4):813-6. doi: 10.1007/s10552-013-0155-7.

37 Cunnane SC, Hamadeh MJ, Liede AC, et al. Nutritional attributes of traditional flaxseed in healthy young adults. Am J Clin Nutr. 1995 Jan;61(1):62-8.

38 Rizos EC, Ntzani EE, Bika E, et al. Association between omega-3 fatty acid supplementation and risk of major cardiovascular disease events: a systematic review and meta-analysis. JAMA. 2012 Sep 12;308(10):1024-33. doi: 10.1001/2012.jama.11374. Review.

39 Grant WB, Schuitemaker GE. Health benefits of higher serum 25-hydroxyvitamin D levels in The Netherlands. J Steroid Biochem Mol Biol. 2010 Jul; 121(1-2):456-8.

40 Holick MF. Vitamin D: evolutionary, physiological and health perspectives. Curr Drug Targets. 2011 Jan;12(1):4-18. Review.

41 Autier P, Bonio M, et al. Vitamin D status and ill health: a systemic review. The Lancet Diabetes & Endocrinology. 2013 Dec 6; doi:10.1016/S2213-8587 (13)70165-7.

42 Rush L, McCartney G, et al. Vitamin D and subsequent all-age and premature mortality: a systematic review. BMC Public Health. 2013 Jul 24;13(1):679.

43 Zheng Y, Zhu J, Zhou M, Cui L, Yao W, et al. (2013) Meta-Analysis of Long-Term Vitamin D Supplementation on Overall Mortality. PLoS ONE 8(12): e82109. doi:10.1371/journal.pone.0082109.

44 Pramyothin P, Holick MF. Vitamin D supplementation: guidelines and evidence for subclinical deficiency. Curr Opin Gastroenterol. 2012 Mar;28(2):139-50.

45 Food and Nutrition Board, Institute of Medicine. Vitamin B12. Dietary Reference Intakes: Thiamin, Riboflavin, Niacin, Vitamin B6, Vitamin B12, Pantothenic Acid, Biotin, and Choline. Washington D.C.: National Academy Press; 1998:306-356.

46 Stabler SP, Allen RH. Vitamin B12 deficiency as a worldwide problem. Annu Rev Nutr. 2004;24:299-326. Review.

47 Lindenbaum J, Healton EB, Savage DG, et al. Neuropsychiatric disorders caused by cobalamin deficiency in the absence of anemia or macrocytosis. N Engl J Med. 1988 Jun 30;318(26):1720-8.

48 Food and Nutrition Board, Institute of Medicine. Dietary Reference Intakes for Thiamin, Riboflavin, Niacin, Vitamin B6, Folate, Vitamin B12, Pantothenic Acid, Biotin, and Choline. Washington, DC: National Academy Press; 2000.

49 Bor MV, von Castel-Roberts KM, Kauwell GP, et al. Daily intake of 4 to 7 microg dietary vitamin B-12 is associated with steady concentrations of vitamin B-12-related biomarkers in a healthy young population. Am J Clin Nutr. 2010 Mar;91(3):571-7.

50 Dangour AD, Allen E, Clarke R, et al. A randomised controlled trial investigating the effect of vitamin B12 supplementation on neurological function in healthy older people: the Older People and Enhanced Neurological function (OPEN) study protocol [ISRCTN54195799]. Nutr J. 2011 Mar 11;10:22.

51 Butler CC, Vidal-Aluball J, Cannings-John R, et al. Oral vitamin B12 versus intramuscular vitamin B12 for vitamin B12 deficiency: a systematic review of randomized controlled trials. Fam Pract. 2006 Jun;23(3):279-85.

52 Koyama K, Yoshida A, et al. Abnormal cyanide metabolism in uraemic patients. Nephrol Dial Transplant. 1997 Aug;12(8):1622-8.